CW01456835

The Genki Self Health Guide:

Improve your Body and Mind with Traditional Oriental Medicine

JOHN DIXON

First published in 2019

Copyright © 2019 John Dixon

John Dixon has asserted his right to be identified as the author of this work under the
Copyright, Design and Patents Act, 1988

All rights are reserved. No part of this publication may be reproduced, stored in any form of
retrieval system or transmitted by any method without first obtaining written permission of the
author.

Disclaimer

All ideas in this book are for informative purposes and is not a substitute for one-to-one
teaching. Seek the guidance of a qualified practitioner when making changes to diet, exercise or
lifestyle. The author and publisher will not be liable for any claim or loss arising due to
following or misuse of the suggestions in this book.

ISBN: 978-1-9998229-1-0

Model: Eitaro Hamano

SILVER NEEDLE PUBLISHING

LONDON

The Genki Self Health Guide:

Improve your Body and Mind with Traditional Oriental Medicine

OTHER BOOKS:

THE TRADITION OF BLIND ACUPUNCTURISTS IN JAPAN: INTERVIEWS WITH SENIOR BLIND ACUPUNCTURISTS AND TEACHERS AT A SCHOOL FOR THE BLIND

FOR MORE INFORMATION

VISIT THE AUTHOR'S WEBSITE AND BLOG

WWW.JOHNDIXONACUPUNCTURE.CO.UK

JOHN DIXON

CONTENTS

FOREWORD

As a practicing acupuncturist in London, England, I have been occasionally asked by patients to recommend a book on Traditional Oriental Medicine so that they could learn more about this field of medicine for themselves.

Whilst looking for a book that I could recommend, I noticed that many of the texts written on Traditional Chinese Medicine tended to be academic in nature and more suitable for the serious student of Eastern medicine. In the end, I could not recommend anything that explained this system of medicine in a way that was simple enough to understand, yet of practical use for the lay person.

For this reason, I have written this book to provide a lay guide on the basic principles of Traditional Oriental Medicine. And to make it useful for the reader, I have included health preservation habits, exercises, food and lifestyle choices.

This book will cover various themes. Firstly, we will look at the theories and principles underpinning Traditional Oriental Medicine such as the concept of Ki or Qi, meaning energy, and specifically the Channel Energetic Pathway system. We will also be looking at the balance of Yin and Yang in the body. This book will provide a brief description of some of the therapies that encompass Traditional Oriental Medicine - acupuncture, moxibustion, acupressure and massage.

Then we will look at basic lifestyle and health preservation habits and practices that can empower us to improve our mind and bodies, such as qigong and meditation, as well as the best ways to use our bodies in daily life to optimize health. I will consider breathing, regulation of the emotions and dealing with physical, emotional and energetic blockades in our bodies.

To finish, I will discuss the introduction and growing popularity of Traditional Oriental Medicine in the West today.

Some of the information in this book will seem like common sense or at times simplistic. However, it is all very practical information. I believe that the more complicated we make things, the less responsibility and control we are able to take for our own bodies and health. Furthermore, the more power we inevitably give to others, especially the pharmaceutical companies.

元気

'Gen-ki'

The title of this book is 'The Genki Self Health Guide'. Genki is a Japanese word meaning 'energetic' or 'full of life'. It is also translated as 'healthy'.

Gen-ki is made up of two radicals - "Gen" meaning 'original' and "Ki", which can be roughly translated as 'energy'. The phrase "O' Genki desu ka?" is often used when inquiring about someone's health and general wellbeing particularly if you haven't seen them for a long time. Its English translation would be "How are things with you? Are you well?"

A Country of Centenarians

In Japan, health is a huge topic of interest as well as a huge industry. It is a country, well known for having a large ageing population and the highest number of centenarians (people aged over one hundred years old). In Japan, a great many elderly people are able-bodied and in relatively good physical health.

Japan is also famous for spreading healthy living practices to the West, such as Shiatsu (finger pressure massage), Zen-meditation and Macrobiotics.

The Japanese diet is well known around the world with the import of popular foods like sushi and sashimi. These delicacies are low in saturated fats, high in fish oils and recognized to be beneficial for the body. It is in this spirit, that I use the word 'Genki' for the title of this book.

I trained in Chinese and Japanese systems of acupuncture and spent some time living in Japan. As a result, I have been greatly influenced by Japanese culture. In this book, I will discuss Chinese medicine, although there will be a special emphasis on traditional medicine from Japan. It is for this reason that I use the term 'Traditional Oriental Medicine' rather than the more commonly used terms such as 'Traditional Chinese Medicine' or 'Traditional Japanese Medicine'.

INTRODUCTION

The Age-Old Question of Health

The topic of health and longevity has been a central issue for humans and civilizations for thousands of years. This was also true for the ancient Chinese Emperors.

The first Chinese Emperor Qin Shi Huang, the creator of the famous Terracotta army, launched an obsessive search for the Elixir of Life. Unfortunately, he wasn't successful and died at age 49.

Other Chinese emperors did not fare so well. In the 'Twenty-Four Histories,' a record of the ancient Chinese dynasties, there were records of other emperors who died from consuming various *elixirs*, which contained deadly substances such as arsenic or mercury. Being healthy was dangerous business.

One of the main reasons why these Emperors were so obsessed with immortality was because things like status, money, fame and power count for nothing without good health to enjoy them. After all, what is the use of all those concubines if you are too sick to enjoy them? Nothing has really changed since then.

There have been times when matters of health were left only to doctors but with the advent of the printing press, the internet and the sharing of information now made possible, it is easier than before to take more responsibility for our own health especially by adopting daily healthy life practices.

Ironically, it is the people with more physically demanding lifestyles and simple, yet adequate diets, that enjoy better health and longevity. Many of us have come across the sprightly 70 or 80 year old who works a physical job and lives on a simple diet. My father is one such example who in his late 70's still mows lawns and gardens for a living. He also lives on a simple diet of fish, bread, porridge and vegetables, grown himself on his London allotment.

Excessive leisure and abundant food can actually be synonymous with poor health. We need only look at King Henry VIII, who in his 50's suffered from obesity, gout and other health afflictions as a result of his life of excess. And herein lies the clue to good health. Good health is about moderation, regular physical exertion and a balanced diet.

In the modern age, many of us can live like kings and emperors. Except, instead of servants, we have labour-saving devices to cook our foods and wash our clothes. We don't need to farm our own food, but only pop into a local supermarket and pick it off the shelves. And magically, we have a variety of foods available to us in abundant quantities. We have elixirs aplenty - a wide range of pharmaceuticals to treat all types of conditions from headaches to depression.

Yet, with this wide range of options, we do not all have perfect health. Far from it. We are missing some pieces of the picture, such as the simple habits of moderation. And there are things we need to be doing in our daily lives as a counterbalance for these modern day lives of plenty.

How many people are aware that if they took 30 minutes a day to do some deep breathing, some light stretching and a little meditation, their physical and mental states could improve and become more stable? High blood pressure lowered, stress levels reduced, sleep and general wellbeing improved.

If more fresh foods were eaten at optimal times of the day with less consumption of processed, junk or frozen foods - digestive complaints like constipation, flatulence and acid reflux could be reduced or eradicated. A lot of pains and aches we suffer from are sometimes the result of faulty living practices – things that if we took the time we could correct ourselves rather than need to swallow a pill.

Listening to the wisdom of the body

The body is a marvelous self-regulating entity, although sometimes it is too perfect because when we treat it badly, it quickly plays up with symptoms and discomfort. We get symptoms of *dis-ease*.

Often, our first course is to shut down our warning systems with drugs like aspirin or repeated courses of antibiotics. But this is akin to removing the red alarm bulb and switching off the siren when the alarm-signal starts flashing then assuming the problem is fixed.

Minor symptoms are our bodies way of showing us that we need to correct certain aspects of our lives. Our bodies are very simple. They need only for us to do and give them what is needed to function better.

In short, our bodies require the following:

1. Regular movement - using our bodies as they were designed to be used.

2. To release tension and ensure a smooth flow of Ki-energy in the body

3. To acknowledge, respect, express and balance our emotions.

4. To balance external activity (yang) with quiet periods of down-time (yin).

5. To eat good quality nourishing foods. To eat an adequate quantity - not too much, not too little. To find pleasure in simple foods and to enjoy and appreciate what we eat.

6. To find a purpose in life (the concept of ikigai), to do fulfilling work and to take care of our financial needs and obligations.

7. To have balanced relationships with family, friends and co-workers and contribute to the society we live in.

In this book, I will address these factors.

To begin with, I will discuss the fundamental basic principles and theories of Traditional Oriental Medicine – yin yang, qi or ki and the Channel system of energy. It is necessary to have a rudimentary understanding of these concepts in order to make sense of the advice and exercises I cover in this guide.

CHAPTER ONE

THEORIES AND PRINCIPLES OF TRADITIONAL ORIENTAL MEDICINE

Attempting to Explain a Different Model of Treatment

There are some unusual words and symbols associated with Traditional Oriental Medicine. A few of these words have been adopted into popular culture such as Yin and Yang, or Qi / Ki energy.

If you practice martial arts, love Kung Fu movies, follow macrobiotics or have an interest in Oriental philosophy or healthcare, you may already be familiar with some of these concepts. However, for the average Westerner, it is not common knowledge.

During an acupuncture treatment, I am aware that the procedures I follow are quite unusual. For example, a person may come in with a headache and I would palpate the outer sides of the feet for tender points and insert a needle there. Or a person may complain of depression and I would palpate the lower abdomen. Occasionally, a person may state "but my stomach is fine".

When you have an understanding of the Oriental theories and its unique map of the body, you would understand that the outer sides of the feet connect to the sides of the head and also that in some systems of acupuncture and shiatsu, abdominal diagnosis is a key part of diagnosis for checking weaknesses of the body, which can be a cause of depression.

A different model of medicine

With Traditional Oriental Medicine, we are using a different model of medicine with different theories, diagnostic methods and treatment techniques. They may seem strange, but they have been practiced for thousands of years.

Acupuncture is constantly developing and every person who practices it or who receives a treatment becomes a part of that process. This is a healthy sign of a dynamic medical system that has continued to grow and spread from its beginnings in Feudal China approximately 5000 years ago to the industrialized and technologically advanced modern cities of today.

The theory of health in Traditional Oriental Medicine is based on several concepts. In this book, I will look at a few of them. In particular, I will discuss:

- The balance of Yin and Yang in the body.
- The flow of Ki or Qi (energy)
- The Channels – a network of energy Channel pathways in which the Ki-energy flows.
- Factors that restrict the flow of Ki in the Channels that impact on our health.
- The status of the emotions and desires and their impact on our health.

Other factors that are deemed important are the seasons, the climate you live in, the foods you eat, the presence of pathogenic factors, the work you do and other external factors such as family, conception and birth, accidents, stresses and daily habits. For more information on these, visit my website.

気

Ki / Qi

Ki (Japanese) or Qi (Chinese) is a word that correlates to the concepts of life force, energy or prana. In this book, I will use the two words - Ki and Qi interchangeably, although they mean the same thing.

In Chinese medicine, there are different types of Ki-energy in the body with different functions. One of the most important types of Ki energy flows through the body along a network of energetic Channel Pathways, also known as Meridians. This Ki powers the functioning of the organs and bodily processes and keeps the body operating smoothly.

This type of Ki energy is unsubstantial and cannot be measured by standard scientific tests. However, it can sometimes be felt by the finely attuned senses of an experienced practitioner. Also sometimes by the patient receiving treatment and by people who do energy practices for a long time, such as qigong or meditation.

The importance of a smooth flow of Ki-energy

The smooth and harmonious flow of adequate amounts of Ki energy in the body ensures the body is in good health and the internal organs are well functioning.

If Ki stagnates in a part of the body, it can lead to pain such as a frozen shoulder or an arthritic joint. If the supply of Ki flow to an organ or in a Channel is insufficient, it causes weakness. For example, if our digestive organs – stomach (and spleen), and intestines has a lack of Ki, we can suffer from poorly digested food, diarrhea, bloating or gas. If we have too much Ki in one part of our body such as the head, we can get headaches or migraines. Traditional Oriental Medicine is about ensuring a harmonious flow of Ki energy in adequate amounts.

The condition of Ki flowing in the channels can be ascertained by interpreting the quality of the radial artery wrist pulse (using a specialist pulse diagnosis technique) and by palpation of the Channels along the muscles of the body. Manipulation of Ki can be carried out with acupuncture needling, moxibustion therapy, which I will describe later, or massage on the acupuncture points. Or by carrying out specific exercises like qigong.

Acupuncture needling has an effect on Ki. It either gathers and strengthens it, or moves or disperses it. A smooth flow of Ki leads to better health and bodily function and is one reason why people who practice the energy exercises – tai chi, meditation, qi gong, or yoga for many years appear younger, more flexible and healthier into their later years. Their muscles are more pliant and loose allowing a smooth flow of energy circulation in the body and internal organs.

During acupuncture treatment, either needling or palpation, the flow of Ki may be perceived by the patient or practitioner. Such sensations may be a feeling of movement flowing along parts of the body like a tingling sensation or electricity-like feeling. These sensations are an indication that the energy of your body is being activated, but it is not necessary to feel these sensations for a treatment to be effective.

Modern day living encourages Ki stasis

Modern day life does not encourage a smooth flow of qi in the body. For example, many modern jobs restrain the Ki. Some jobs involve spending 8-10 hours a day sitting down, be it an office worker or a HGV driver.

People who do these kinds of jobs can suffer from back ache or shoulder stiffness because the energy in the back and lower limbs is not encouraged to move. The muscles are held in a constricted pose for many hours and energy gets stuck in the upper body causing shoulder stiffness or it gathers in the buttocks, leading to weight gain in this area.

The antidote to this is movement, to get the energy moving through these Channels. It does not need to be the higher intensity type physical exercise like going to the gym and lifting weights. It can be simply going for walks in the park, swimming or dancing. Even housework or gardening work can make huge differences if done regularly.

Another factor that can stagnate the flow of Ki is the emotions, which I will discuss later.

Yin and Yang

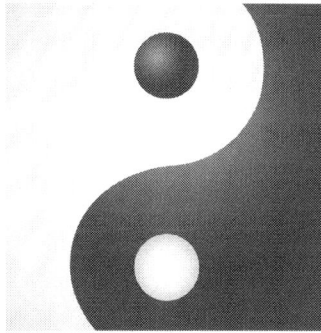

Unique to Traditional Oriental Medicine is the concept of yin and yang and particularly how it relates to sickness in the body. At its heart, Yin and Yang is a simple, yet sophisticated way of understanding the human body and the universe.

Yin and yang may be described as complementary opposites that comprise everything in the universe and the human body. It refers very simply to the balance of energy in the universe and within ourselves.

An understanding of yin and yang can deepen the Chinese medicine practitioner's understanding of disharmony in the body. In short, when the balance of yin and yang in the body is normal, good health is ensured. When it becomes unbalanced, disharmony and sickness occurs.

The classical yin yang symbol is a circle made up of black and white with two dots within each part. The symbol is found on the South Korean flag and is often seen in magazines, on posters, clothing and tattoos. The black represents yin. The white represents yang. Within yin, there is an element of yang and within yang there is an element of yin.

Yang is attributed with the qualities of expansion, light, heat, fire, growth, activity, the sun, the outer, the male, the sky or heavens. Yin is attributed with qualities of darkness, cold, water, rest and rejuvenation, the moon, the inner, the female, the earth.

Yin and yang are present in everything and are relative to each other. Within yin, there are elements of yang and within yang there is yin. For example, the daytime is considered yang and yet different times of the day may be considered to be more yin than yang. The afternoon when the sun is at its brightest is said to be most yang, but the evening just before dusk as it starts to become darker can be said to be the most yin within the yang.

Yin and yang are not meant to be concrete qualities or polar opposites. They are simple human expressions to describe a universe that is in constant fluidic motion. It is a simple yet elegant expression.

Yin and Yang in the Human Body

The concept of yin and yang can be applied to parts of the human body, which can be divided into yin and yang areas.

For example, the skin is considered yang compared to the deeper internal organs, which are yin. The upper body is considered yang as it is close to the heavens and the lower body is yin as it is closer to the earth.

The blood and body fluids is considered yin as it is thick and full of precious substances, whereas the oxygen and breath is yang as they are relatively insubstantial. The front is considered yin and the back is yang for if you consider that man evolved to walk in an upright state, the back would have been exposed to the sun (yang) in prehistoric man, who may have walked hunched over in a manner closer to walking on all fours.

The internal organs are also divided into yin and yang. The organs which are classed as holding vessels (stomach, large and small intestines, bladder and gallbladder) are considered yang. The organs which hold the precious substances and bodily fluids like the kidney, heart and liver are considered yin. The lungs are also classed as yin although they are the most yang of the yin organs.

Yin and yang can become imbalanced in various ways. For example, yang energy has a tendency to rise in the body. In some cases, there may be too much yang in the upper part and not enough below. This can manifest itself as recurrent headaches or chronically stiff shoulders where the energy gets stuck above. At the same time, a person may suffer from cold hands and feet or a weakness in the limbs.

Over-thinking, worry or pensiveness causes the qi to stagnate or knot. One example of this is the 'butterflies in the stomach' sensation, when a person feels anxiousness in the pit of their gut, when faced with a worrying situation. Anger causes a person's energy to go upwards, causing a red face or a propensity to lose their temper easily. Both worry and anger can lead to disturbed sleep and nightmares.

Insomnia is another example of too much energy above. A person cannot fall asleep – their minds are too active (yang) and they think excessively. At worst, a person starts to worry that if they can't sleep they won't be productive the next day, which becomes almost a vicious circle because as you think more and more, it becomes difficult to sleep.

In this situation, it is almost impossible to think yourself to sleep, because what needs to be done is to bring the energy back into the body and away from the head. There are various exercises that can help such as meditation or deep breathing exercises. These practices are yin in nature and can help counterbalance the excess yang (overthinking).

In some people, the lower energy centers are weak because all the yang energy is directed away from them, which can show itself up as dull low back pain, poor digestive function or excessive urination. Painful swollen joints as in the inflamed state of rheumatoid arthritis and various inflammatory conditions like colitis, hepatitis or ulcers, also indicate an excess of yang energy in the sick part of the body.

Inflammation, or heat, is yang. However, in people with these conditions, there may well be another part of the body or organ system which is too yin or deficient and which may need to be addressed in order to rebalance the yin yang energy.

There are various ways we can help ourselves if we feel we have an imbalance of yin and yang. Firstly, we need to take a scrutinising look at our lifestyle and its possible influence on our health.

If we are office workers and spend a huge amount of time sitting and using the eyes and brain looking at a computer screen, the yang energy will be stuck in our head for 8 hours a day. Also our muscles will be deprived of a fresh flow of blood and yin energy because we hold them unnaturally in a sitting posture.

The antidote to this is that when we finish work, we should divert the energy back into the body by walking home or going swimming or to a gym, yoga or tai chi class to counteract the energy flow. Alternatively, if you are a manual worker – a bricklayer or gardener, then the yang energy has been used a lot in the body and to rebalance the yin yang flow, more relaxation exercises – such as seated meditation or a nap or reading a book in the evening can be beneficial.

If we notice a part of the body seems excessively cold or weak – for example the lower back or belly, then a hot water bottle held against it can bring the energy back there. If our limbs or back muscles feel stiff in a dull (deficient way), then going for a massage can be beneficial as someone else helps generate yang energy for you. These are simple ways to redistribute the Yin Yang energies of the body.

This is a basic introduction to yin and yang in our bodies. But yin and yang is a broad topic and goes deeper to include things like the effect of the changing seasons on the body, the stages of sickness, the stages of growth from childhood to old age, the effects of different foods on our bodies and much more.

Acupuncture

Acupuncture is a system of medicine whereby specific points on the body called acupuncture points or acupoints, which run along special energy Channel pathways on the body are stimulated by needles in order to achieve a beneficial effect in the body. We will discuss the Channel pathway of Ki later. The needles used in the modern age, are very fine, sterile or disposable, usually made from stainless steel but can be made from gold or silver. Gold and silver needles are usually used for non-insertive techniques.

Needles can be inserted into the body and retained for a period of between 10 to 45 minutes. In the Japanese tradition of acupuncture, a needle may be touched and briefly held against the skin in a technique known as *contact needling*, until a change is perceived by the practitioner. Acupuncture needles are thinner than hypodermic needles so needling is relatively painless. Anything from a single needle to up to 40 needles can be used in a single treatment.

Though it may sound painful and the idea of needling puts a lot of people off going for acupuncture with memories of having injections or dental work done, the process of having acupuncture can be a very pleasant and relaxing experience.

The needles are relatively painless. Sometimes, they are not even felt when being inserted. I find that once the needles are in, the patient enters a high state of relaxation – a kind of meditative zone, where they can reflect, relax and connect with their bodies. It is in this state that healing can occur.

Treatment results can vary. Sometimes results can be immediate or effects may occur in the next few days. Occasionally, a condition may be aggravated and then will settle down again, particularly if the problem has been entrenched for some time or if an over-treatment has occurred. Some conditions require several treatments for a change to be effected.

Moxibustion

Acupuncture treatment also utilises another type of therapy, which is quite powerful in its own right. Moxibustion or 'moxa' is the practice of burning mugwort (*Artemisia vulgaris*) on various acupoints, on tense muscles or in other areas of the body to create a beneficial effect. Receiving a moxa treatment can be very relaxing and produce a pleasant warming effect. Moxa can be used to bring warmth and energy to weak deficient points and areas or it can move areas of stagnation. There are two fundamental ways of using moxa – *indirect* and *direct* moxa.

Moxibustion also comes in several forms. For example, there is a processed natural form which can be rolled in tiny rice-grain sized cones and then burnt on specific acupoints. Or larger cones which can help to move stagnant energy. These larger cones are not burnt all the way down but are removed after they are half burnt, so protecting the skin.

Moxa can be applied indirectly in a cigar form which projects a gentle heat onto the point. A moxa box is sometime used – a wooden box containing burning moxa, which is then placed on the lower abdomen or lower back and which projects warmth and heat into these areas. It is particularly useful for low back pain or digestive weakness.

There are smokeless variations for rooms where ventilation is a problem or an electronic moxa device is available and sometimes used by blind acupuncturists in Japan. A heat lamp may also be used to simulate the warming effects of moxa. Patient safety is paramount when carrying out moxibustion and though there is a risk of burning or scarring, moxa is safe when carried out by a trained practitioner.

Acupuncture and Moxibustion

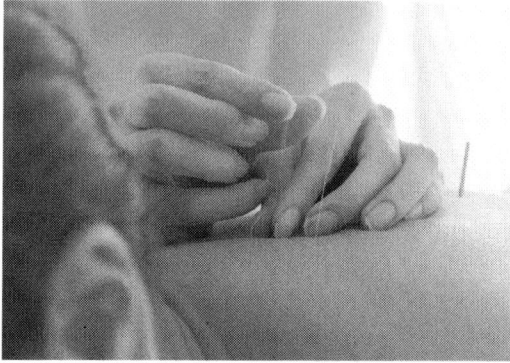

Acupuncture: Insertion of sterile filiform needles into specific acupoints in the body

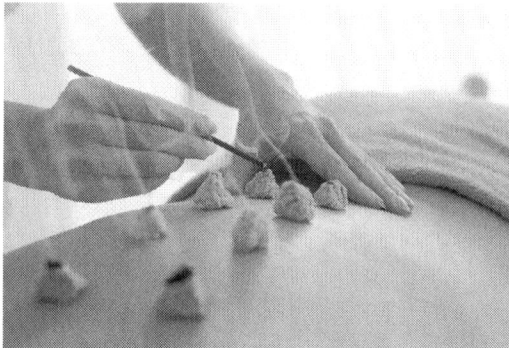

Japanese moxibustion or "moxa" cones. Burning of mogwort (Artemisia vulgaris) on acupuncture points

Other Therapies in Traditional Oriental Medicine

There are other therapies that make up traditional Chinese and Japanese medicine. These include massage, herbal medicine and the health preservation exercises such as Tai Chi and Qigong. I will discuss Qigong and massage in a later chapter. Herbal medicine is a vast subject which I do not practice and so I would recommend anyone interested to find alternative sources of information.

CHAPTER TWO

THE CHANNEL SYSTEM

A patient may visit an acupuncturist with a problem in one part of their body such as their lower back. The practitioner may treat directly the affected area with needles or moxibustion but then the patient may also be somewhat mystified when needles are put into the back of the calf muscles or on the outside of their ankles or in their foot.

The reason is that there is a Channel or energetic pathway that leads from the lower back down the back of the leg and to the foot. In this example, it is called the 'Bladder Channel' and gets its name because this particular Channel branches off internally and passes through the actual bladder organ (over which it has a special influence).

This Bladder Channel also travels upwards to the head and ends at the eye, meaning that points along this Channel can be used to treat eye problems, bladder weakness, back pain, sciatica or ankle pain.

This is a simplified example of how the Channel system of Traditional Oriental Medicine works. These Channels, also known as *Meridians*, are pathways where the Ki travels through the body.

The Channel Pathways

The Channel system is a series of energetic pathways, which traverse the body from the toes and finger tips, through the limbs and torso, and into the head. These pathways travel superficially along the surface as well as deep through the muscles, flesh and the internal organs.

In total, there are 72 Channels in the body, although in standard acupuncture treatment, 12 main Channels are used alongside 8 *extra* or *special* Channels, which behave more like reservoirs for energy. The Channels are an interconnected whole and there are many connections and branches between them, although certain Channels tend to have closer relationships to others. It is on these Channels that the acupuncture points or *acupoints* are located.

In modern Chinese medicine theory, the 12 major Channels are named after a particular organ which they travel through and have a predominant effect upon. So, for example, the Liver Channel is so named, because it passes through the physical liver organ. The Kidney Channel passes through the kidneys. The Gallbladder Channel passes through the gallbladder.

In this book, I have capitalized the organs when I refer to them in the Channel meaning of the word. When I refer to the physical organ itself, I have used lower case letters. For example – 'the *Kidney* Channel passes through the *kidney* organ.'

However, the Liver Channel and the liver organ are still two separate entities. If an acupuncturist says – 'Oh, your Liver Channel is weak' - this does not mean the liver organ is weak. It means the energetic pathway of the named 'Liver Channel' is weak or out of balance. It does not mean you should go out and have liver function tests. These tests will most likely not find anything abnormal.

What is does mean is that any bodily functions that comes under the realm of the Liver Channel may be affected. For example, the Liver Channel opens into the eyes, so eye problems may be related to weak Liver qi flow. It affects the reproductive system in women by encouraging the liver to store blood, meaning that menstrual difficulties may be related to the Liver Channel energy. It controls the sinews, which means it is implicated whenever we have muscular pains.

Acupuncturists can treat an organ directly if it is sick or under-functioning, but there will be an emphasis on rebalancing the Channels.

Acupuncture Channel Network

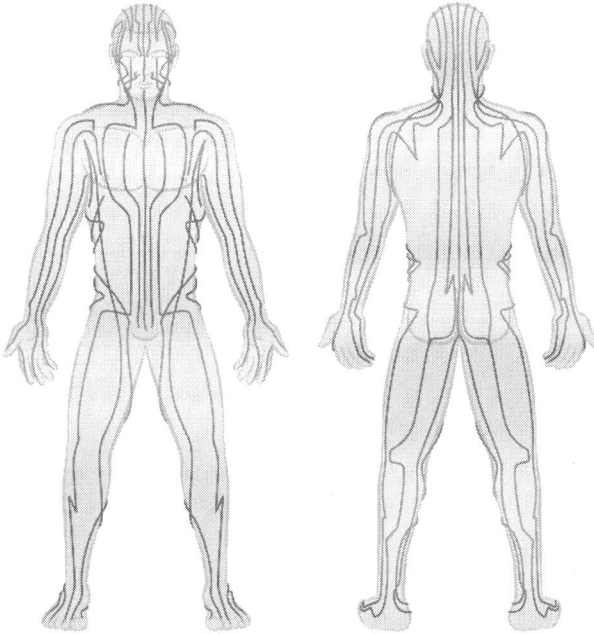

Diagram showing the major Channel networks in the body, on which the acupuncture points lie.

In the case of low back pain, the Bladder Channel that passes through the lower back also travels through the back of the knees and the outer sides of the ankles. An acupuncture treatment may involve needling the knees and outer ankle because it will have an effect on the whole Channel and the lower back.

The Small Intestine Channel, which passes through the shoulder, also goes to the hand. So, for shoulder pain, a point on the side of the hand will be used.

A more recognizable sign of the Channel system can be seen in heart problems. For example, a common medical observation in people suffering a heart attack is a tingling feeling that runs down the arm to the little finger.

From a Traditional Oriental Medicine point of view, this pathway exactly follows the Heart Channel which connects from the heart organ, passes through the axilla (armpit) and travels down to the little finger. Sometimes, it is often a related Channel that is the source of the problem and not the main Channel that runs through the area where the problem is located.

Think of your body as a country. The Channels are the road networks and the Ki energy are the vehicles travelling along them. The Channels are made up of different types of roads – small lanes, duel carriageways and motorways with numerous junctions and smaller roads linking everything up.

With an adequate number of cars (Ki energy) driving safely and orderly, traffic can flow smoothly. However, if an accident occurs, there are roadworks, or there are simply too many cars, then traffic seizes up for hours (causing a stagnation of Ki). In this case, people get stressed, drivers use other roads, which in turn clogs them up. Then supplies or deliveries are delayed and people cannot get back to their homes and become even more stressed. The country (you) becomes out of balance. The body is the same.

There are main Channels, which connect with each other in a circuit with smaller Channels such as the Luo or Divergent Channels. If the Channels are in good condition and the flow of Ki is harmonious, the body works well. But if there are problems, the flow of Ki stagnates and poor health occurs.

Ki flows through the Channels in a circuit running through each of the 12 main channels at different times during a 24-hour cycle. Using current scientific equipment, it is difficult to detect the existence of the Channels. However, some research shows that there are electrical differences in the areas of the acupuncture points on a Channel compared to non-acupuncture points.

It is also possible to develop sensitivity to the Channels and to actually feel changes along them. I have heard that some Taoist monks are even able to see the pathways with their third eye, although I have not met anyone who is able to do this yet. But what I have seen in clinical practice is people with areas of pain, or a rash on an arm or limb, that seems to follows exactly the Channel pathway.

I have also seen huge depressions at acupuncture points on Channels that are related to their health problem, where your finger literally sinks into a dip. When people are needled, they may feel a tingling or flowing sensation that follows the trajectory of a Channel pathway when asked to explain the sensation.

Acupuncture Points

Acupuncture points or 'acupoints' are special openings on the Channel pathways where the Ki energy is accessible and can be manipulated. There are some theories, where it is believed that if all the acupoints are opened up and clear, good health is experienced. In Traditional Chinese and Japanese Medicine, these points are needled or stimulated with finger pressure or moxibustion to rebalance the bodies energies. By stimulating these points, the flow of Ki can be normalized resulting in better health.

The acupuncture points have been mapped up and can be seen in diagrams. During the Song dynasty (960 AD to 1279 AD), a bronze man was fashioned in China with 657 holes in his body corresponding to the acupuncture points. The bronze statue was then covered in wax and filled with water, and acupuncture students were then tested by inserting a needle into the correct location of the acupuncture point. If they succeeded, water would flow out of the hole.

There are even possibilities that acupuncture was known in the West thousands of years earlier. Otzi the iceman is a 5000-year-old mummy discovered in the Otzal Alps in Southern Austria with 50 tattoos on his body that archaeologists believed may have corresponded to acupuncture points.

In modern physical therapy work, many of the acupuncture points correspond to the trigger points. Trigger points are tight spots in the fascial tissues surrounding the skeletal muscle, believed to be the focal point of a muscle in spasm, which when treated can help relieve pain in the muscle.

The acupuncture points on the Channels are known as openings where the Ki of the Channel flows close to the surface and can be accessed by finger pressure, burning of moxa, or acupuncture needles.

There are 365 classified points. 365 corresponds to the days of the calendar. The Chinese were influenced by nature and the seasons and this set number corresponds to the number of days in the year. However, there are many more non-classified points than this. All of the main points have been mapped out and can be located by following very clear anatomical descriptions.

Active acupuncture points

Another factor is that some acupuncture points are active and dynamic and others will be inactive. They change their quality according to the condition of the body in health and disease.

To give an example, in someone who has severe stomach problems, such as ulcers, or has had digestive problems for many years – if we palpate the Stomach and Spleen Channels – which relate to the digestion, we may find that some of the acupuncture points feel very weak or are painful to the touch. As we stroke along the Channel to a known acupuncture point, our fingers may drop into an obvious depression, or may stop at a soft or weak area where the acupuncture point is. All of these findings indicate that the acupuncture point and associated Channel is 'active' and indicates disease or disharmony in the body.

Any particular reaction along the pathway, like a perceptible weakness, a dullish pain, sharp pain or depression tells us that this acupuncture point is active and needs to be treated. The observation that acupuncture points can change their qualities from one patient to another does make it hard to carry out standard research studies except for conditions like osteoarthritis of the knee and back, where disease tends to be fixed in one place.

The active points are not always the same for everyone. As there are various Channels running through any particular problem area, it is always necessary to feel for the most reactive points, because these are the points which manifest disease.

Take the Lung Channel for example; the Lung Channel influences the lungs, nose and skin. If the flow of energy is weak in this Channel, certain symptoms like cough, colds and breathing problems like asthma may occur. Skin problems like acne may also occur. To diagnose and treat problems on this Channel, an acupuncturist may select acupuncture points along the Lung Channel.

If the Stomach or Spleen Channel is weak, symptoms related to digestion such as loose stools or abdominal pain may occur. Treatment will involve balancing the energy in this Channel by treating acupoints. A commonly used acupuncture point is the Stomach-36 Point, which is shown in the chapter on acupressure later on.

Another example is shoulder stiffness. The Small Intestine Channel passes through the shoulder area and any kind of pain in this area usually indicates a stagnation of energy or blood in this Channel. Treatment may involve moving the flow of qi in this Channel using points on the shoulder with either needles or burning moxa on it.

If above, treat below. If left, look right

A common practice in modern Oriental medicine treatment is to insert needles into the site of a physical problem. For example, if someone suffers headaches, typically several needles may be inserted into the scalp or around the temples. This would be classed as a local treatment. This kind of treatment makes a lot of sense to a patient. The problem is in my head, so treat my head.

Other times in acupuncture treatment, it can be better not to treat the problem locally i.e. at the site of the problem.

The ancient classical texts make a recommendation that if the problem is above, then treat below. If it is below, then treat above, if the problem is on the back, then treat the front.

It is also possible to get good results by treating the right side if the left side is diseased and vice versa. One practical application of this is where there is a patient with a cast over one arm or may even be missing a limb and suffering from phantom nerve pain. You cannot directly treat that arm, but it is possible to treat the relevant points on the opposite arm.

The channels are a mirror. Treating one side will affect the other. You may have to explain this to the patient, who will probably think you weren't listening when she told you her right arm was broken not the left.

One rationale is that you want to move the energy. One part of the body has too much energy. Another part has too little. One side is healthy. One side is diseased. Therefore, we should balance the sick side with the healthy side. We should balance the excess side with the deficient side. The body is a connected whole and we should try not to compartmentalize it.

It is tempting to think that the problem is in my right leg, so only my right leg is sick. Or the problem is in my knee so my knee is sick. The problem in my leg may be caused by the digestive system. The knee pain could be caused by a problem in the back or hip. Some problems may even be caused by the emotions.

Disease is dynamic

Another issue, is that very rarely is there only one Channel affected with a health problem. Quite often, two or three Channels will be in various states of weakness or deficiency. The human body is dynamic – ever changing as we age.

Disease in the body is also dynamic and will change its location and nature over time as it runs its course. Some imbalances in one Channel over time will start to affect other Channels manifesting as new diseases and symptoms.

The body becomes a landscape. Everything is connected. Even the smallest sign or symptom will have some relevance. It is up to the acupuncturist to take all this information and evaluate it and see how it makes up the bigger picture of your body and your life.

In this way, true integrative healing can occur. This is something that also everyone can do for themselves if he or she has an understanding of the nature of the human body.

Yin and Yang and the Channel System

The Channels should also be considered in the context of Yin and Yang. Channels are also classified as Yin and Yang. The Channels that pass through the 'Yin' organs – the heart, kidney, spleen, lungs and liver are classed as Yin meridians. Channels that pass through the Yang organs – stomach, intestines, gallbladder and bladder are classed as Yang organs.

On observation, the yang Channels tend to be on yang areas of the body such as the back and on the outer part of the limbs, whereas the yin Channels are on yin areas of the body such as the front and inner part of the limbs although there are a few exceptions to the rule. All of the yang Channels meet in the head which is the most yang area of the body.

When it comes to sickness in the body, the acupuncturist may observe imbalances between the yin and yang channels in the body which are severe enough to manifest symptoms. The job of the acupuncturist is then to balance the channels accordingly.

Typically, if energy is excessive in one channel, there will be a related weakness in another channel or another part of the same channel. The trained acupuncturist can assess if this is the case simply by palpating the channels and feeling for weak or hard areas along the Channels.

Applying these principles to the body

At this point, we have looked at some of the theories and principles behind Traditional Oriental Medicine. In the next few chapters, we will look at how it can benefit our everyday lives and contribute to our long-term health. Different aspects of health will be talked about under the following sections:

- Movement and activity: Using the body in daily activity and ensuring a smooth flow of Ki

- Stress and Tension

- Breath

- The Benefit of Meditation

- Emotions

- Food

- Massage & Acupressure for Self-health

- Our Relations to Others/Family/Society

- Dealing with Life Challenges

- Purpose of Life

CHAPTER THREE

MOVEMENT AND ACTIVITY: USING THE BODY IN DAILY ACTIVITY AND ENSURING A SMOOTH FLOW OF KI

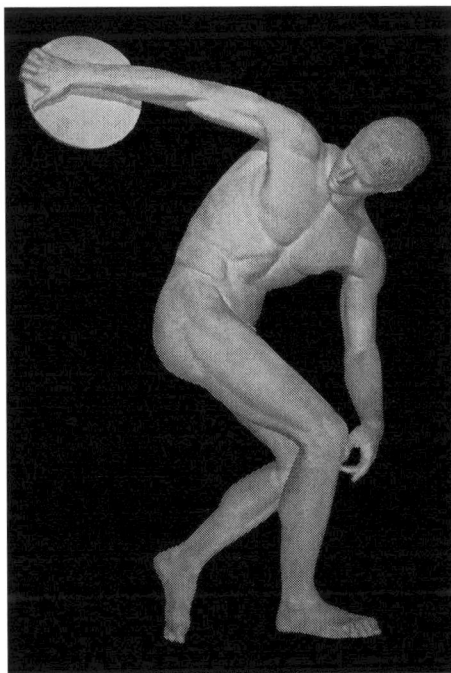

The Discobolus of Myron

This image of the ancient Greek statue - the Discobolus of Myron shows the muscular toned physique of a young athletic male throwing the discos. The ancient Greeks were particularly interested in the human form and made many statues showing vigorous strong male figures or sensual and fertile women. Essentially, they show the human form in its perfection.

For centuries, various civilisations have developed different physical ways of developing and training the body from sports to combat training, swimming, running, fighting, martial arts training or bodybuilding. But for everyday people, it has been centuries of daily physical work such as farming, building, carpentry, gardening, building work, laboring jobs, soldiering, housekeeping and cleaning, which has kept our bodies, slim, strong, hardy and relatively resilient.

Right up to the 1950s in the UK, people were mostly engaged in physical work although the trend has gradually reduced as labor saving devices and white goods have become common and jobs have become less physically orientated in the West.

Geoff Pike, a qigong master now in his 80s, wrote about how physical activity has an important impact on our health in his book 'Chi: The Power Within':

> "As a general rule, the strongest and fittest among us are those who work outdoors. But the number of such people is finishing in the face of the rapid takeover of air-conditioned, computerized, mechanical labour-savers....
>
> We have all admired the professional ski instructor, swimming, tennis or football coach, the gold pro or gym instructor who is well past forty and still going strong. Consider a person who has spent a lifetime outdoors engaged in some kind of physical work. Chances are he is stronger and sounder than his counterpart behind a desk, closeted in air-conditioning and artificial light".

The most common human movements that make up daily human life are:

- Lying
- Sitting
- Standing
- Walking
- Running
- Getting up / getting down / bending

Daily life and activity should involve a balance of some of these movements if we want to stay supple. At different stages of our life, we favor certain motions more than others. For example, younger children never seem to tire of getting up, crawling or bending over. If we watch older children at play on a grassy field, we see they favour spontaneous running and tumbling.

Adults may practice controlled running (marathon training) and sometimes controlled tumbling (as used in some martial arts). Elderly people may favor walking over running but if they are sport focused, they may enjoy running. Those suffering from illness, convalescing or restoring their energies after a heavy day of physical work will favour lying or sitting.

We may notice that some types of mindset are related to specific activities. For example, people who are depressed or apathetic may spend a lot of time sitting, lying or sleeping. Certain jobs require excessive amounts of standing such as guards or security. All of these movements shape our body structures accordingly. As regards shape – out bodies adapt to the demands placed on them and may develop or under-develop certain muscle groups with some muscles becoming shorter and less flexible or longer and more flexible depending on the need.

If we are active, our muscles become more toned, developed or fuller. If we move very little, our muscles become flaccid or reduce in size. People who sit a lot may find more weight gain around the bottom area.

The Floor Culture of Japan

I lived for a few years in Japan, and one of the first cultural lessons you learn is to always remove your shoes when entering someone's home. One of the main reasons for this is that in Japan there is a large traditional floor culture, where people sit and lie down on the floor instead of in chairs or on sofas, and no one wants to bring rubbish from outside into your living space, particularly to where you are in close proximity to the floor.

Though some Westerners view the habit of removing shoes at the door a curious habit bordering on strange, I recall a time when I stepped in dog-poo (unfortunately a common problem on British streets) and without realising, bought it into a friend's house. I spent an embarrassing 20 minutes helping my friend clean it up with a bucket of hot water and soap and repeatedly apologized.

I look back on this incident and think just how easily it could have been avoided if we had a similar culture where shoes are removed at the doors of people's houses. Whenever I visit someone's house particularly for a home acupuncture visit, I always offer to take my shoes off.

In Japan, rather than sitting on sofas and chairs, family members sit on the floor. In the center room of the home is the 'kotatsu' – a low square table which has a heater built inside it and which family members can put their feet under for warmth during the winter months. The floor is not carpeted as in western homes.

Instead either wooden floorboards or a bamboo-type matting called tatami is used, which is firm yet soft to sit on. Meals are eaten around the kotatsu and family members can socialise and sit around it when friends come around. People will also sleep on these tatami floors on futon mats, which are rolled up and stored during the day until it is time to go to sleep again. In this way, even the process of going to sleep and waking up involves physical activity twice a day as you roll out and fold up the futon and sheets.

Floor culture has many benefits. Firstly, repeatedly getting up and sitting down becomes a form of exercise in itself. We are forced to use all our muscles every time we get up and down with nothing to use as support other than the floor. Contrast that with large sofas into which we flop into and which support our bodies in a semi lying state. Though they are comfortable, they gradually weaken our muscles because even though it looks as though we are sitting upright in a chair, in actuality we are closer to lying down.

Sitting in a sofa becomes an extension of sleep whereas sitting on a flat surface is true sitting. Sofas are wonderful inventions. After a busy and tiring day, there is nothing more relaxing than flopping into a sofa with a beer and snacks and a TV programme, but it would be more beneficial to our postures and muscles if we were to sit cross-legged on our sofas in order to stretch out the hips especially when watching TV, reading or talking on the phone.

One of the main problems with sitting in sofas is that we tend to bend our heads forward which restricts the chest and our lung capacity and which encourages poor breathing habits. The back of our necks and shoulders are overstretched eventually weakening them and the muscles in the front of our bodies go tight leading to postural imbalances such as the excessive forward head posture.

Modern day sitting and its effects on the musculature

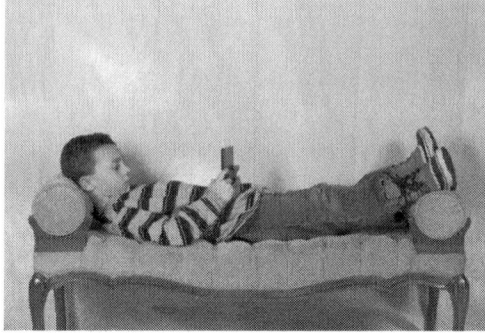

Slumped sofa sitting shortens and tighten the chest muscles

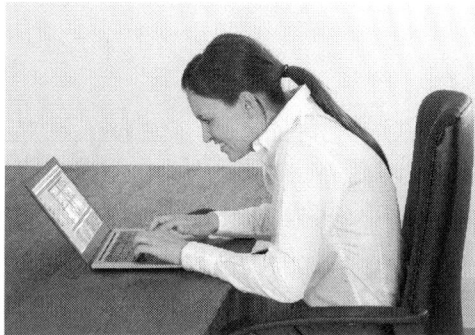

Office workers frequently suffer from low back pain, or shoulder stiffness caused by excessive sitting and leaning over a computer screen.

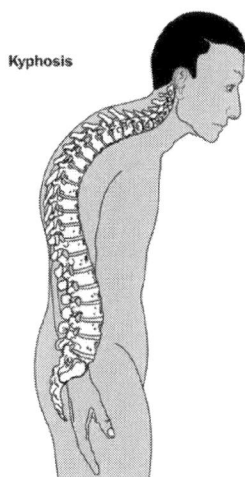

Above: Ingrained poor postural habits can lead to kyphosis or the forward head posture.

Posture and Personality

How we use our bodies on a regular basis affects our personality and values. For example, we see it in members of the forces who are taught to stand with an erect carriage and walk straight with daily parades and marching practice as well as to speak loudly and clearly without hesitation leading to a firm, albeit less emotive personality.

In contrast, if we watch a tabloid talk program like the Jeremy Kyle show, the UK equivalent of the Jerry Springer show, we see many of the participants with slumped bodies, dull expressions, scruffy clothes and appearance and quickness to anger. Their postures betray their attitudes and mindset.

If we observe the ease at which they lose control of their emotions, particularly anger, and the ease that they give in to their desires - mainly sexual affairs with neighbours or relatives along with their absent or dis-interested parenting and lack of responsibility to even their own families let alone the rest of society, we see very clearly how their appearance and posture clearly reflect their personality and attitude to life.

In the UK, the numbers of people with these attitudes is increasing particularly in the home counties and old manufacturing towns, where industry and jobs have gone with nothing to replace them with.

Excessive Slumping

This is a habit that can be created very early on in life and can be difficult to stop once set. Children, who are naturally a burning force of energy are taught to sit still at desks for several hours a day. On the plus side, they learn discipline and the habit of study and concentration.

However, study must be balanced with adequate daily activity such as sports and play to burn off the extra energy children are naturally endowed with. In the modern age, children are far less active than previous generations. A lot of home activities encourage excessive slumping such as playing video games and watching TV.

The problem is partly confounded by fear of letting children free to play outside, particularly in big cities like London in case something happens to them. This continues throughout most of childhood and extends into early adulthood as children go to college, university and then onto company jobs that involve sitting and staring at screens. Other types of jobs require sitting for prolonged periods of the day such as drivers, check out assistants or telesales.

The Western chair is actually poorly designed for our body. The back rest encourages people to slump, which gradually leads to a weakening of our back muscles and leads to a shortening of our hamstrings.

Often the head protrudes forward to look at screens, which over-stresses the upper shoulders and neck muscles and can lead to stiff shoulders and constricted pectoral muscles, restricting our lung capacity.

This means that our bodies do not breathe in the higher levels of oxygen, which our bodies are capable of, nor are they able to remove waste carbon dioxide as effectively. The modern way of sitting is actually quite harmful for our bodies and can gradually lead to back pain, shoulder stiffness, neck pain and sometimes headaches.

The antidote to poor sitting habits is to practice beneficial sitting habits and cultivate new habits. Adopting the floor culture habits of the East may help but if this is too alien, then some of these habits can be adapted to suit our modern lifestyles. For example, we could position ourselves cross-legged whilst sitting on sofas instead of sinking into it to help stretch out our hips.

Obviously, it is not possible to do this at most jobs and so time can be set aside at home to cultivate these habits. 10 to 20 minutes every day at home can help the body to redesign and correct its muscular imbalances. For sitting, the two best postures to adopt are cross-legged sitting and seiza.

Cross-legged Sitting

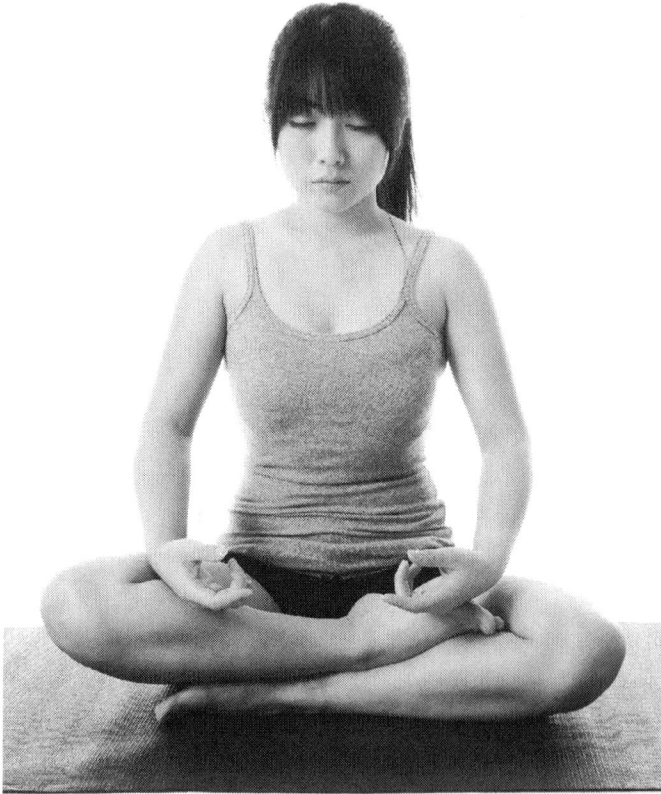

The simple cross-legged position is a common pose which helps open up the hips and lower back and stretches the outer aspects of the legs. Many children can sit naturally in the cross-legged position until they are trained in sitting in chairs. The cross-legged position is one of the healthiest ways to sit and it is no coincidence that it is the same form of sitting practiced in Indian yoga or meditation.

The lotus position is derived from the basic cross-legged position. Sitting cross-legged opens up the hips and releases the muscles of the waist and lower back by passively stretching them. It also encourages the body to hold itself upright on its own accord which strengthens the lower back muscles especially if whilst sitting in this position you consciously make an effort to straighten your spine and hold yourself upright.

After weeks of regular practice of sitting cross-legged, improvements to posture can occur - you can stand taller and feel your posture is more upright. Unfortunately, years of sitting in chairs can actually make it very difficult to sit cross-legged without discomfort or pain. The reason is that our bodies are adaptive machines. They conform, adapt and change themselves accordingly to whatever forces we subject them to.

Our bodies adapt quite well to slumping in chairs but when required to sit on the floor suddenly all manner of aches and creaks as well as pins and needles are regular occurrences. Even worse, is that if we try to force ourselves to sit cross-legged in an attempt to get used to this pose quickly and gain its benefits (an ego trick), it can lead to muscular or joint pain.

This kind of discomfort should always be acknowledged. If pain occurs then it is better to stop sitting in this way. The mantra – 'no pain, no gain' does not refer to muscular, tendon or joint pain because otherwise real physical damage can occur and take time to recover from. Sometimes a slower approach is better.

For some people, the body can be retrained back to sitting cross-legged, though it may take months, even years and should be done gradually. You may also find that after a few minutes of sitting in this way, you feel tired. This is because your body has to use specific muscles in your lower back and hip in ways it is no longer used to.

This tiredness is an indication that your muscles are getting a *work-out* and that they are being trained. In a sense, this is similar to the kind of working out when you go to a gym and do a series of exercises, which after a while feel tiring, but which over time can lead to increased strength. The difference is that this 'work out' is more *internal* and less dramatic. There is less involvement of the ego.

People will go to the gym and lift heavy weights in order to build larger biceps, but few will think to practice sitting straight in order to build better upright posture. Yet, time and again, people will admire upright posture in a person far more than large biceps as it makes a person look more confident and attractive.

Over time and with regular practice, you will find it easier to hold this sitting position. If pins and needles occur, then get up and move your legs for a few minutes and then resume again the sitting posture. It is beneficial to aim to sit for ten to fifteen minutes a day in this way as long as it is comfortable.

Seiza Sitting

正座

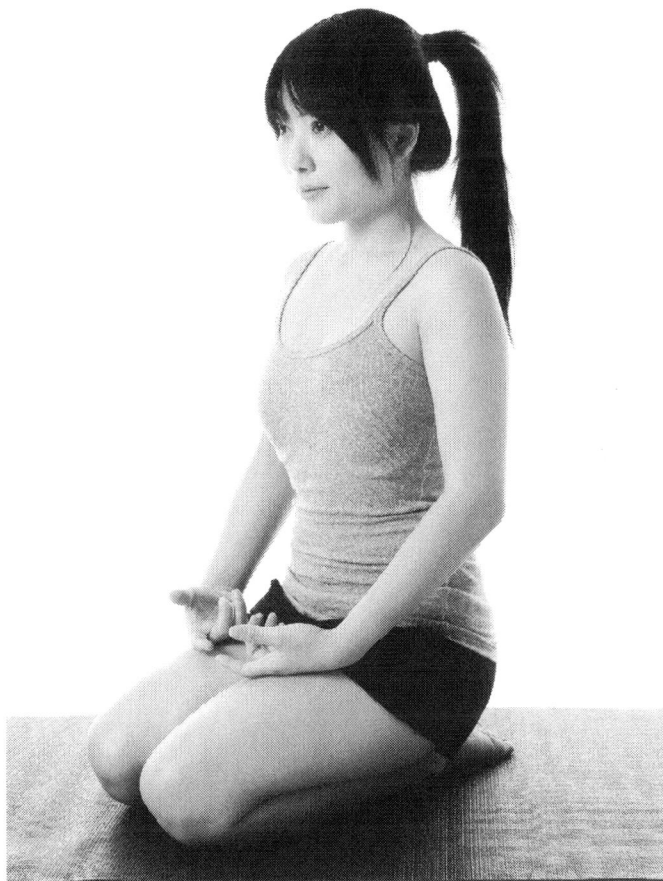

Upright or correct sitting

Seiza is a form of sitting where you sit with an upright back and your legs folded under your bottom. The Japanese word seiza translates simply as 'upright' or 'correct sitting'. It is often used in certain martial art practices such as aikido, partly because from this pose it is possible to quickly stand up from the seiza position in readiness for action. It is also used in meditation and breathing practices and in performing ceremonies and rituals.

Sitting in seiza with the spine upright frees up the ribcage making deep breathing easier. By gently tucking the chin in, the spine is lengthened, which opens up one of the central energetic Channel pathways - the *du mai,* which runs along the spine of the body. Meditation can be experienced deeply if carried out in this position.

From an acupuncture perspective, sitting in seiza position opens up the Stomach and Spleen Channel pathways, which corresponds to digestion. This is because these channels run along the anterior aspects of the legs, which are stretched and opened out allowing Ki energy to flow more smoothly. Also, the acupoints along this channel are further stimulated by being pressed into the floor as you sit in this pose. This stimulation and opening up of these channels is beneficial for digestion.

Again, many people find it very difficult to sit in this position unless they have been conditioned for it. The use of cushions particularly under the bottom which raises the height of the torso and puts less pressure on the back muscles may be advisable as it also takes the pressure off the legs.

Over time, the muscles in the legs will gradually lengthen and you will be able to sit in this position but it should never be forced as otherwise damage can occur. Again, if pins and needles occur, stand up and move around to gets the circulation flowing and then resume.

The art of seiza sitting has a positive effect on our personality by helping to impart a stoic mentality. By keeping the back straight and conditioning the body to endure some minor discomfort, it makes the body and the mind stronger over time.

Wisdom of the Babies Body

In the first 6 months, babies will develop their stomach muscles and be able to raise their legs. They will be able to hold their neck upright. Around the age of 10 months, babies are able to sit upright with legs out or slightly crossed. They are able to do a full forward bend even put their toes in their mouth. Babies constantly use all the muscles of their body, twisting, bending, standing up and falling. As a result, their bodies are loose and supple.

There are many adults (myself included) who cannot do some of these movements. And yet, at some point in our life, many of us would have been able to do this. It's a flexibility which many adults tend to lose unless they practice certain physical activities like dance training, gymnastics or yoga. The adage – *'use it or lose it'* is quite fitting. If we continue to sit as babies sit, we may well keep that flexibility, but as adults, we generally don't.

The Flow of Energy in the Body

We talked earlier about the ancient Oriental concept of Qi/Ki. The major energy channels of the body flow through the muscles. If a muscle is tight and shortened, it means that there is a poor flow of Qi/Ki through the Channel in that muscle, which also means there will be a restricted circulation of blood and lymph in that muscle or area of the body.

If the muscular restriction is very bad, there may be tight aching muscles. If there is restriction in a joint, we may find that arthritis occurs. In the case of arthritis, it may possibly be reversed if it is not too advanced.

Daily Movement

The healthiest and longest living people on the plant are those that incorporate some kind of physical activity into their daily routine. There are some people in their 80's, 90's and even 100's who still perform daily physical work. These days with the many advancements in healthcare, people can survive into their 80's and 90's, but their health and quality of life may not be so good. There is a difference between being in your 80's and bedbound compared to being in your 80's and living an active and independent life.

In a study in the National Geographic magazine on areas of the planet that held relatively larger amounts of healthy active centurions, various factors of longevity were identified – one of which was that some of these people still worked. Daily physical activity conveys many benefits.

Gardening, fishing, house-cleaning on a regular basis, yoga or tai chi, walking or any kind of activity can keep your muscles loose and supple, open up the joints and help calm the mind. As humans, we need to be busy and have a purpose to our lives otherwise lethargy, laziness and boredom can creep in, which can be toxic to our physical health and mental wellbeing.

Retirement age is usually around the age of 60 to 65 in the West and there is a mental expectation to slow down and become 'old' at this point. People do indeed do this, which implies there is a mental aspect to becoming old. Some people do not and it may be the case that you can think yourself *old* or think yourself *young* and your body responds accordingly as some people remain physically very active well into their 70's and do not see themselves as old.

Some people may still have a good many year's work left in them after retirement age. My father is a good example. As my father approaches his 80's he is still very physically active - regularly doing gardening work, maintaining an allotment growing all his own vegetables and going backpacking on hiking trips in South East Asia once a year just like a gap-year college student. A lifetime of activity and hard physical work has conditioned him in this way.

One example of this was years ago when I went trekking in the Himalayas with him. At the start of the Annapurna range, we had to walk up a very steep long winding set of stone steps – it seemed like 1 to 2 miles straight upwards.

As a young man in my 20's and supposedly at the peak of health, I had thought myself fit at the time. However, within minutes I was panting, wheezing and sweating like a pig. I must have looked like I was about to collapse as our guide insisted he carry my back pack for me despite my objections. I felt embarrassed at being the only one struggling.

My father, who was in his late sixties at the time had no problems whatsoever because even though this was his first-time trekking, his body was already so well-conditioned from a lifetime of physical activity, he could do this relatively comfortably. Fortunately, after a couple of days, I became more accustomed to the trek, but this beginning was a humbling lesson for me.

There are several well-known Japanese acupuncturists who are still working well into their 70's and 80's. For acupuncturists in Japan, there is no concept of retiring at 65. In fact, at that age, some of them may feel they are only just beginning to get good. Work or activity keeps them young. Humans are at their best when they are occupied with useful daily tasks.

With the growing number of baby boomers reaching retirement age with a great many of them still in good physical health, that plan to spend those retirement years living in a villa in Spain, going on cruises or relaxing with day time TV or at the local pub is like a double-edged sword.

CHAPTER FOUR

THE BENEFITS OF REGULAR WALKING

The human body is designed to walk long distances. Our ancestors walked much further than we do today. The further back in time you go, the further our ancestors walked in an average week. Obviously, one reason being that there were less transport options available. Some of the greatest civilizations were built on the ability of its citizens to be able to walk hundreds of miles.

The ancient Roman soldiers marched throughout Europe and North Africa carrying their supplies and armour. They were physically strong and well-disciplined and conquered much of Europe, the Middle East and North Africa on foot. Alexander the Great's armies travelled on foot from Greece and to the outskirts of India on foot and back again.

The British army on foot was able to win significant battles in India in the 1800's, leading to its eventual colonization. Then on foot, they took on Napoleons armies marching through Portugal, Spain and into France. Napoleon's armies were able to march on foot from France and take the city of Moscow. A hundred years later, Hitler's armies in motorized cars couldn't get that far.

Humans are quite well adapted to travelling long distances on foot. Yet today, most people will walk less than a mile a day sometimes not even fifty meters. Primitive man may have walked miles a day foraging and hunting. In some African and South American Rainforest Tribes, men walk for hours foraging or hunting making them lean and strong. Walking has a great many benefits to human health.

As our transport systems became more advanced, humans had less need to walk. Cars, trains, buses, elevators, escalators as well as supermarkets, washing machines, water pipes and heating systems at home means that people can now be carried everywhere and that they no longer have to travel distances to obtain food, clean water or to wash clothes.

These are all great things as the purpose of technology has always been to free up human labour. The downside is that we walk less and sit more, which weakens our bodies. The ability to walk as a baby signifies the first sign of independence in life and the loss of ability to walk in old age signifies the first sign of dependency on others again.

We should be grateful for the gift of walking and take the chance to practice more. There are simple ways to get more movement in our daily life. For example, we can get off a stop early on the bus or train and walk the rest of the distance. We can walk up and down stairs and escalators instead of being carried. One of the greatest ways is to go hill walking. In Japan, I enjoyed walking up mountains and relished the inevitable muscle aches for the following days.

10,000 Steps

In Japan in the 1960s, Dr Yoshiro Hatano and a team of researchers were investigating the new trend of rising obesity in the newly affluent Japan. The increasing number of overweight people were worrying the Japanese even back then. They found that if people walked 10,000 steps a day, people would be healthier and thinner. At the time, people were walking on average 3,500-5000 steps a day.

Hatano developed a pedometer called a 'Manpo-kei' (10,000 step meter) to encourage people to achieve this. Today, these guidelines are encouraged by the World Health Organisation (WHO) and National Health Service (NHS) in the UK although it is advised that this number is adjusted depending on your physical condition. Elderly and people with chronic diseases are advised to walk less than this and some children could be advised to walk more than 10,000 steps.

On a side note, I once attached a pedometer to my 18-month-old boy just before letting him loose in a soft play area. After 30 minutes of walking, running, climbing and jumping, he had cracked up an impressive 1,000 steps. Like a lot of children, he is lean and fit.

Generally, walking is as effective a way of burning calories as running the same distance and requires less exertion. As a teenager growing up in the 1950s my father told me that most women were nearly all lean and physically attractive as the norm. One of the reasons was that people moved and walked more then.

Even long-distance travel has changed dramatically. For example, a taxi picks us up from home and drops us off at the airport, where we queue at the check in, walk to the terminal, walk on the plane, then sit down for 12 hours to arrive at the other side of the planet. Then we walk off the plane, queue and pass customs, walk to the taxi rank or coach stand which takes us direct to the hotel to check-in. Finally, we take the elevator and walk a few feet to our hotel room. We have travelled 5000 miles yet walked less than half a mile during that journey.

Walking in Ancient Rome

If we return to the west, the walk or gait was of considerable importance in the ancient Roman world and gave an indication of your character and importance. In the Book 'Walking in Roman Culture', O'Sullivan, discusses how the ancient Romans consciously cultivated an art of walking, which was not *"just a way of moving through space, but also a performance of identity"*. He also talks about the belief of something called *'the rule of the gait'* - how your way of walking actually defined who you are.

For the elite Romans, walking was more than a method of going from one point to another. It was also seen as a way to reflect or to converse with others in conversation. The manner of walking - not too slow like a woman and not too fast like a slave - reflected your social position and importance. Walking was itself an art form. Who would think today that walking could have such a deeper meaning?

If we take a few minutes to sit and observe a busy street and watch the different people walk past, we can observe all manner of walking and gaits which can actually tell us something about the personality of the people. How a person holds themselves and how they walk tells us about how they see and think of themselves in the world. Also, if we take a few minutes to look at how we walk, it can tell us something about ourselves.

I like to walk slow and steady and to think on things as I walk. I dislike being made to walk to a quick pace which reflects my own independent mind and a tendency towards a relaxed contemplative life.

After reading this, take some time to look at how you walk and what does it tell you about your personality? Even experiment with different styles of walking and take note of the different feelings and mindsets that may be associated with different ways of walking. It is best to do this while walking of course.

Benefits of Walking

We take the power of walking for granted. It is only when we lose that ability, that we appreciate its benefits. Walking signifies independence and freedom. Walking is one of the simplest exercises and is probably the best exercise to build our physical power, health and to purify our minds.

In 'The Power of Qi', Geoff Pike wrote:

"The heart of a lion cannot be supported on the legs of a chicken".

Leg strength is important for longevity. We take our legs for granted but as we get older one of the biggest problems we face is mobility – weak legs and balance issues.

Regular walking gently builds up muscle endurance and strength in the lower body. It is also good for gently building up bone density. Osteoporosis (a lack of bone density) is a problem that we can be affected by as we age or if we suffer from illness, especially for women. One way to counteract loss of bone density is with weight resistance exercises, but these exercises are not always suitable for everyone.

Walking is a low impact exercise and can be less damaging on the joints than running. However, if someone is in poor health or is recovering from illness, walking may not be advisable or if someone has balance issues and is at risk of falls then this type of exercise may not be suitable as there can be a significant risk of injury or harm.

By walking, blood and lymph is pumped and circulated more readily around the body as we contract and relax the various muscles of the legs through the process of walking. This is more important in the legs as our movement stimulates the lymph vessels to push the lymph fluids and its wastes upwards against gravity to be processed.

By walking, we encourage this pumping action of the calf muscles which help clean out the body internally and can help drain excess fluids in the legs and prevent varicose veins. As we walk, we tend to breathe deeper naturally, steadily enthusing our bodies with life-giving oxygen and helping to remove CO_2 wastes.

Walking opens up our spine in contrast to excess sitting which exerts pressure and tension on it. Our feet contain many muscles which often get neglected. Walking helps to massage and stimulate these muscles. Daily walking for 30 minutes can help to tone and stimulate our feet.

The scientist, Taro Abo talks of the usefulness of walking to help balance our emotions in his book – 'The Only Two Causes of All Diseases':

"By living as a human, there always can be bumps in the road and at some points in your life, there may be a time where you get continuously irritated and lose the balance in your lifestyle.

When you get that continuous feeling of irritation and you are not cooling down, please remember to take a walk for a change. By walking, the lower half of your body is stimulated so the unbalanced blood flow rushing into your brain will be resolved. As a result, you will naturally regain your cool demeanor".

So we see, that walking is not just only physically beneficial for us. It also helps balance our emotions and can dissipate anger, which is by far one of the most harmful emotions that can affect us.

Reflexology and the Feet

Stimulating and massaging the feet is far more important than we realize. Reflexology is a system of massage whereby areas on the feet also known as 'reflex zones' correspond to areas in the body.

It is believed that problems in the body can show up as physical changes on the corresponding areas on the foot manifesting in ways such as hardened areas of skin, tenderness, painful areas and a buildup of crystal-like substances under the skin which feel very crunchy when pressed. These are called 'crystals' and are believed to be a buildup of calcium deposits.

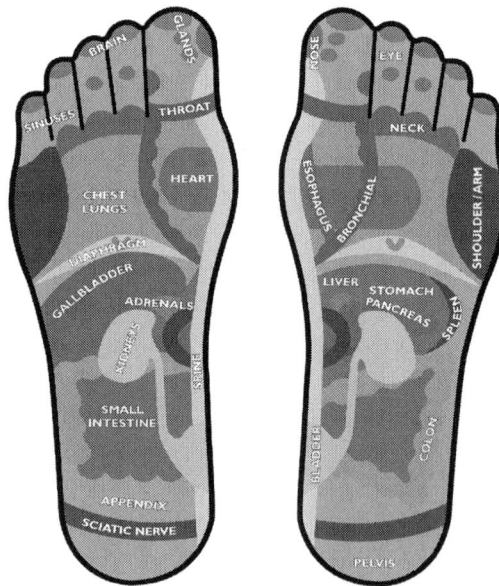

Diagram of Reflexology foot map indicating how specific areas of the foot correspond to different organs or parts of the body.

It is believed that bodily imbalances can be helped by pressing on these 'out-of-balance' areas. Reflexology is also extremely relaxing and it is not unusual to fall asleep during a treatment and to feel calmer and more relaxed after treatment.

There is a Japanese comedy film called 'Maiko Haaan', a movie about Geisha and Maiko. A Geisha is a high-class entertainer and hostess that wears extravagant white makeup and are trained from an early age to play instruments and perform traditional dance. A Maiko is usually a young girl who is an apprentice Geisha.

The actor Sadao Abe plays a company worker who is obsessed with Maiko and it is his dream to be allowed to enter the Geisha quarters in the ancient capital of Kyoto - an honour usually only reserved for very rich, powerful, politicians, company presidents or famous celebrities.

After succeeding at work with a huge sales project that makes a lot of money for his company, his president invites him to a famous Geisha house in Kyoto so his dream can finally come true.

As he enters the building, all Japanese are expected to remove their shoes and wear a special kind of indoor slipper. However, as the doorman takes his shoes from him, he looks at them with a scrutinizing eye and interrupts him suddenly. They have the following conversation:

Maiko Han

Doorman: - "Sir, it's difficult to say this to you but please go to hospital immediately.

Customer: - "What?"

Doorman: - "I've been doing this job for forty years and I can see the health condition of my customers clearly by looking at their shoes".

Customer: - "Hey, don't say scary things to me after I worked so hard without sleep or rest, day and night to get this reward".

Doorman: - "I see… your body is worn out by stress and lack of sleep. I'm telling you this for your own good. Go and see a doctor."

After some argument, his boss persuades him to see a doctor. He goes to the hospital and is immediately admitted.

Doctor: - "There's a hole in your stomach, a urethral stone and herpes virus too! Ah, your body is worn out with stress and lack of sleep"

Customer: - "I worked too hard!"

Doctor: - "Operation right now."

Although this is a comedy, there is some reality in this. Illness and problems can show up in the way we carry ourselves, in our posture and our gait. If we notice that one side of our heel tends to wear away in a specific pattern in all our shoes, it could indicate various imbalances in our pelvis or that one leg may be slightly longer than the other possibly caused by one set of muscle groups in our inner thigh being shorter or tighter than the other side.

Usually, these problems won't cause any obvious health problem, but can indicate an imbalance in our bodies that could be worth addressing early on. A chronic stomach pain can sometimes cause a person to tense or clutch their abdominal area which can cause a person to slightly bend over.

If it continues for a long time, this postural habit can become more engrained. And this is what the holistic healer learns to do. They must be able to see the person from the moment they walk in the door and pick up on all of these signs, because ultimately, it can help them to focus on what is likely wrong and what needs to be corrected in that person.

Basically, the body is a canvass. It shows all of our life's experiences, our traumas, our emotional and psychological experiences – whether they were good or bad, our past medical problems, our constitutional strengths and weakness that we were born with, our attitude to life, our current and past stresses.

The truly enlightened practitioner will pick up on all of this. I am not so talented as to be able to pick up on these, but as we practice more we learn to 'intuitively' detect when someone may have a certain kind of problem or life experience especially if we can keep mental clarity, ignore our own internal voice within and tune in with the patient in front of us.

This is truly a holistic way of looking at the body by seeing it in its entirety and to treat what we see. In a seminar, I attended with John Hicks, a Five Elements Acupuncturist, author and teacher, he recommended an exercise, whereby we imitate the body and posture of a patient or anyone you see to get an inner understanding of that person. However, he warns about taking on the role too much in case you start to develop similar symptoms that this person may suffer from!

For a moment, just stop and watch how you are holding yourself. How are you breathing? Is there any tension or restriction in any part of your body or your face? If there is, what is causing it? We all invariably carry some habits or tensions that become so habitual, we no longer realize it. It is often only when someone else mentions it, do we realize.

Soft feet

In the modern age, we have a greater need for practices like reflexology. In the past, our ancestors would have found their feet were more naturally stimulated in their daily lives. Our feet are designed for wear and some tear. The heels and soles are especially harder and can benefit from walking on hard surfaces as well as walking for long distances.

The ancient Romans wore sandals made of wood and leather, which would have been harder than modern shoes. Walking on harder surfaces or rough terrains inadvertently massages the feet every time we walk on them and allows for the natural stimulation of the reflexology points on our feet.

Today this stimulation is limited – we wear socks all year round, we walk on carpeted floors. Popular trainers are well cushioned to adapt to running on hard concrete type surfaces. The skin on our feet is generally softer and there is less stimulation. Sweaty feet and nail infections are common because feet are not aired out enough. To counteract this, it is possible to buy reflexology slippers in order to stimulate these points on the feet as we walk but they are a lesser substitute for barefoot walking.

A father has never liked to wear socks. Even when working at farm work or construction, he would wear his boots without socks inside. As a result, the skin on his soles was thick. He had strong feet but more valuably, he was robust and healthy.

The downside is that he often annoyed my aunt, because whenever he went to visit her and took his shoes off in her home, the soles of his feet were often not much cleaner than the bottom of his shoes. She often bought him socks for Christmas and birthdays as a hint, which he in turn gave away.

In Japan, a reflexology tool called Takifumi was developed to stimulate these reflex areas on the foot at home and can be practiced by yourself. 'Taki' means 'bamboo' and 'fumi' means 'to step on'. It involves stepping on bamboo (a hard wood-like round plant) to stimulate the feet. It was said to be practiced by the samurai warriors.

It is also possible to buy substitute takefumi or massage boards made of plastic and rubber over the internet.

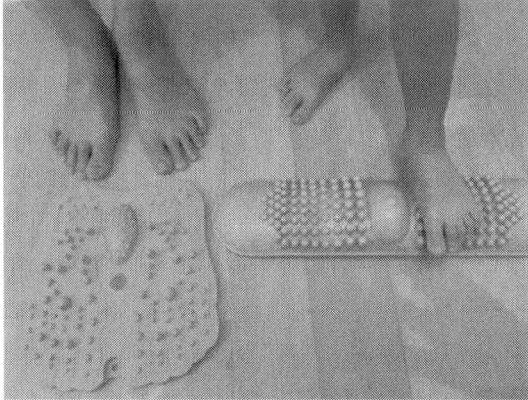

Ready-made Takefumi - Foot Massage boards, that I bought in Japan from a Hyaku-En shop (£1-pound shop).

Some traditional martial arts like karate, judo and aikido carry out their practices barefooted on hard mats. This is partly to limit any damage to other members of the class as shoes can cause more injury to a person if kicked by them, but going barefoot also strengthens the feet.

Recently, the practice of 'barefoot running' has become more popular and has been promoted as being beneficial to the feet. I believe this is only the case as regards running on soft terrains like desert sands or on beaches where the impact to joints is softened. I don't believe it is suitable for running on concrete roads in cities or towns, otherwise injuries can be picked up such as joint inflammation or shin splints.

Most people's feet are too soft to be able to safely run barefoot without injury. Another problem with going barefoot in populated areas is the danger of stepping on sharp objects – broken bits of glass, litter, dog mess or having your feet stepped on.

Overall, one of the best things we can do is to go barefooted at home. If we have wood flooring it is even better. Also take the opportunity to walk barefoot as often as possible in the garden, park or on the beach.

Fire below, Water Above and our Feet

We looked earlier in the discussion of yin and yang in the body at the concept of having *fire below, water above and a cool head'* for health. One way to bring heat down is the Chinese health preservation exercise of soaking your feet twice a day in warm salty water for about 20 minutes each time. Soaking the feet draws heat from the upper body bringing it back down to the feet. This method can also help people who have sleep problems.

There is definitely a correlation between having warm feet and becoming relaxed and sleepy. Anyone who has had a reflexology treatment will be able to tell you that it's quite common to doze off during the treatment. The gentle massage warms the feet.

There are exceptions - for example some Thai masseurs use really strong and painful pressure to stimulate the points, but generally, most reflexology treatments are very relaxing. It's perfect if you have a family member who can rub your feet just before going to sleep.

CHAPTER FIVE

SIMPLE EXERCISES TO OPEN UP THE BODY

In yoga, there are two poses named the cat pose and the dog pose which are full body stretches. Cats and dogs stretch their bodies in similar ways to these poses, particularly after waking, hence the name.

After a period of rest and immobility or after a night's sleep, our bodies naturally want to stretch and open up and if we are in tune with them, our bodies will guide us into performing various stretches of limbs and arms shortly after we wake up after a night's sleep.

Stretching helps warm the muscles up and opens ups areas of the body. For example, the common stretch upon waking, where both arms are pushed upwards and we let out an exhale, helps to naturally open up the chest and shoulders and helps to breathe out stale air from our lungs.

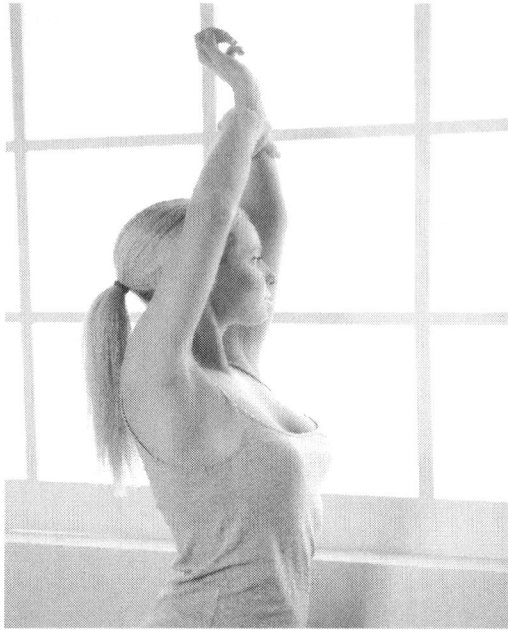

The morning stretch - the body guides us into opening up our bodies

Other people feel a need to stretch the legs outwards and lengthen the hamstrings. These stretches are a wonderful gift because it is the body communicating with us directly as to what it needs. Stretching also helps prevent injuries and pulled muscles by warming up the body and preparing them for movement.

One of the easiest ways to cause a painful pulled muscle or muscle-spasm is by performing a sudden jerky muscle movement with cold muscles – muscles that have not been warmed up adequately. Muscle spasms can take days to recover.

As an acupuncturist, this is a common problem I have been contacted to treat. One way to reduce this risk is to perform daily warm-up routines or stretches lasting 5 to 10 minutes especially if you are doing manual work. These exercises are simple and gentle and I will cover some of them in this chapter. They are also often used as warm-ups in martial arts where strength, muscle flexibility and explosive power is required.

Understand that injuries in martial arts negate the whole point of a martial art. For example, if a highly famed warrior with decades of experience was to suddenly put his back out whilst in the middle of a battle and had to be stretchered out screaming in agony – "*my back my back!*", the Emperor would not be too impressed. Hence there is a need to warm up at the beginning of the day.

A good example can be seen in the final fight scene in the movie 'The Way of the Dragon. The martial art masters Bruce Lee and Chuck Norris prepare to face off against each other in the Roman colosseum. However, before fighting, they take almost a minute and a half to warm up their bodies with stretching. This is quite a long scene for a movie. It provides a level of realism and shows how these two fighter wanted to perform at their optimal best in preparation for the fight. Most martial art or kung fu movies do not include this kind of scene.

Stretching and warming up does not necessarily mean that you will never get injuries but it can reduce the chances of it happening. More importantly - gentle opening-up exercises can promote good joint flexibility and stave off arthritic-type conditions which tend to affect the joints as we get older.

Here are a set of warming up and opening up exercises. They should be carried out gently and in a relaxed manner for 5 – 10 minutes every morning shortly after waking. They encompass the opening-up of all the major joints of the body where our energies can become stagnated and can over time can help improve our posture and gait.

1. Circling the Waist

This exercise gently warms up and stretches the waist, abdomen, lower back and opens up the hip and upper legs. It strengthens the back muscles and can prevent lower back pain when you get older.

- Stand with legs shoulder-width apart. Put your hands on your hips.

- Push your hips to the front.

- Breathe in and move your hips in a circle to the right, and then round to the back pushing your bottom out.

- As you breathe out, keep circling to the left and to the front again.

- Breathe in and repeat three more times. Then reverse direction for four more times.

Circling the Waist

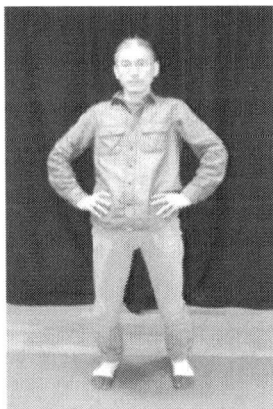

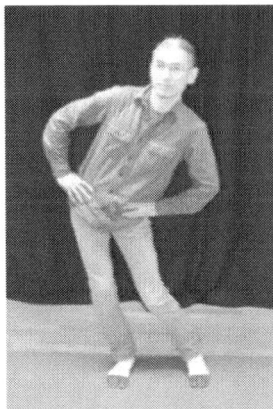

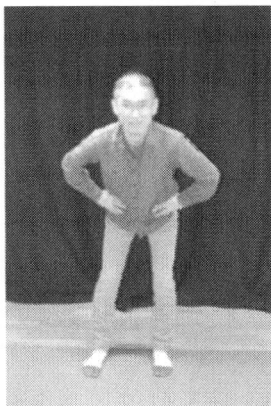

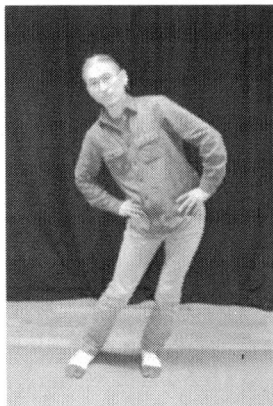

2. Head rolls

This exercise stretches the muscles of the neck, upper shoulder, back and chest. Tightness in these muscles can cause neck and jaw pain and headaches. This exercise should be done in a gentle circular motion, whilst breathing in and out, in a smooth co-ordinated movement.

- Stand or sit straight with your arms by your side.

- Breathe in and gently drop your head forward so your chin is touching your chest. You will feel a stretch in the back of your neck.

- Breathe in and gently circle your head to the right so your ear almost brushes past your shoulder. Keep breathing and circle it to the back, opening up the front of your neck.

- Breathe out and continue rotating to the left and round to the front position again.

- Continue three more times, and then change direction for four times.

Head Rolls

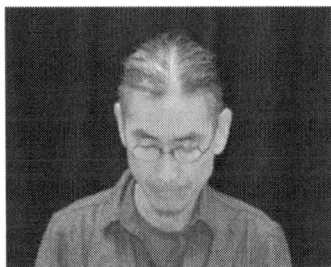 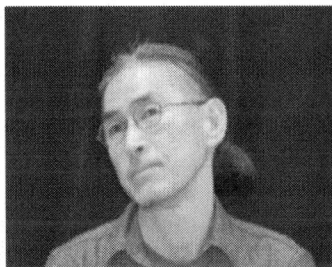

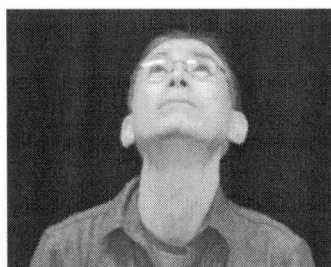 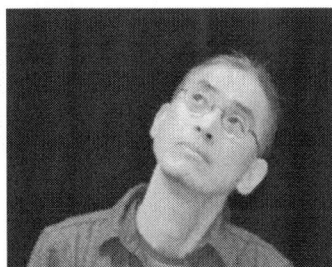

3. Circle the knees

The knees are a joint that need to support the weight of the whole body. Being overweight puts a lot of pressure on this area. These exercises gently strengthen the knees and prevents against knee pain.

- Stand with both feet close together. Gently bend your knees bringing your hips lower and put your hands on your knees.

- Breathe in, and in a smooth circular motion, move your knees to the right and to the back. Breathe out and circle to the left and to the front again.

Circle the knees

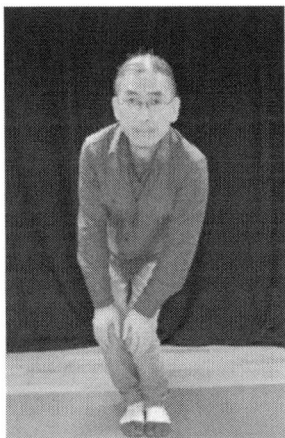

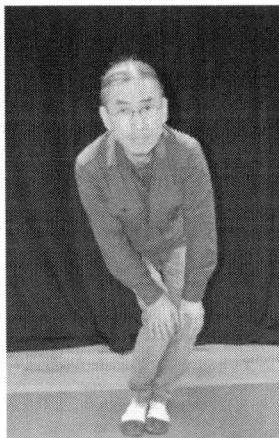

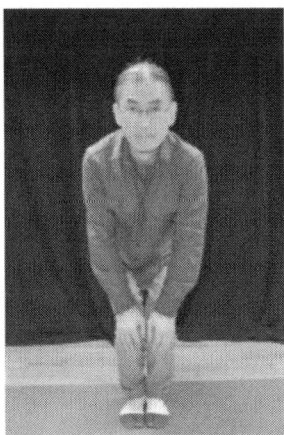

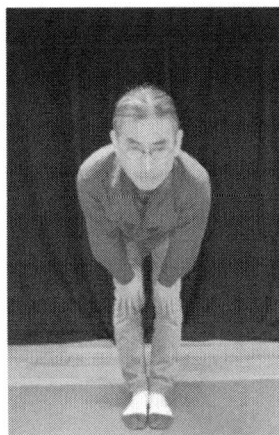

4. Up-Stretch / Reach for the Sky

If you've ever seen a cat stretch its whole body when it wakes up, this exercise has a similar effect. It enlivens your entire spine, arms and legs.

- Stand with feet shoulder-width apart or close together.

- Take a deep breath, and as you breathe out reach your arms to the sky and stretch.

- Hold for thirty seconds and release. Repeat as many times as you want.

You want to stretch the spine and open up the space between each vertebra. People who sit down a lot slumped at desks or in front of computers will have vertebrae that are closed tight together and para-spinal muscles that are weak.

The spinal column houses an important network of nerves and blood vessels. If these are contracted together, their functioning is hindered making us operate less effectively.

When you stretch, use your imagination as though an invisible thread is pulling you up into the universe whilst your feet are being pulled to the center of the earth.

Up-Stretch / Reach for the Sky

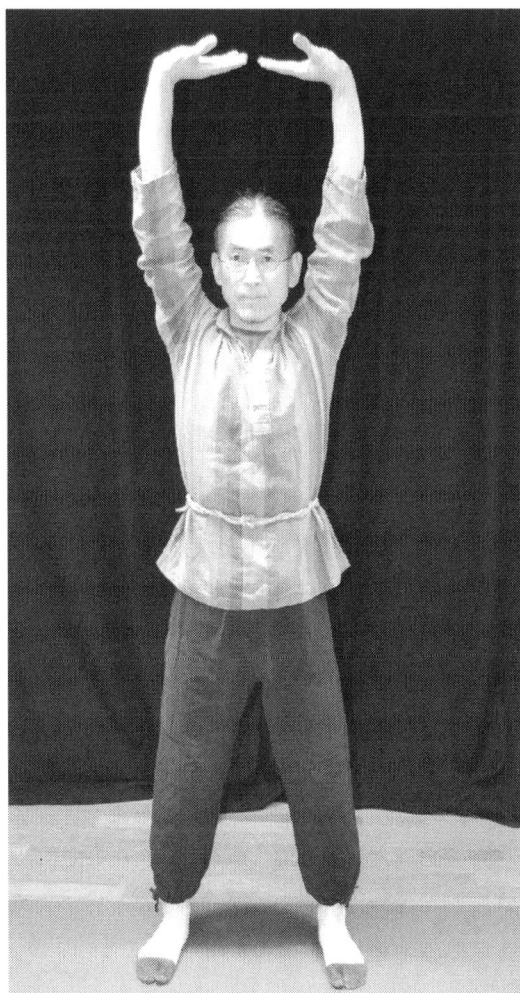

5. Down-Stretch / Standing forward bend

Excessive sitting causes the muscles of the back and hamstrings to shorten and leads to poor posture. The forward bend is one of the best stretches to counteract this.

- Stand with legs shoulder-width apart.

- Take a long breath in and as you breathe out, gently bend forward from the hips and reach for the floor. Keep the back of the knees straight.

- Relax into the stretch and just let it hang. Breathe normally for one to three minutes and gently return to the original position.

Down-Stretch / Standing forward bend

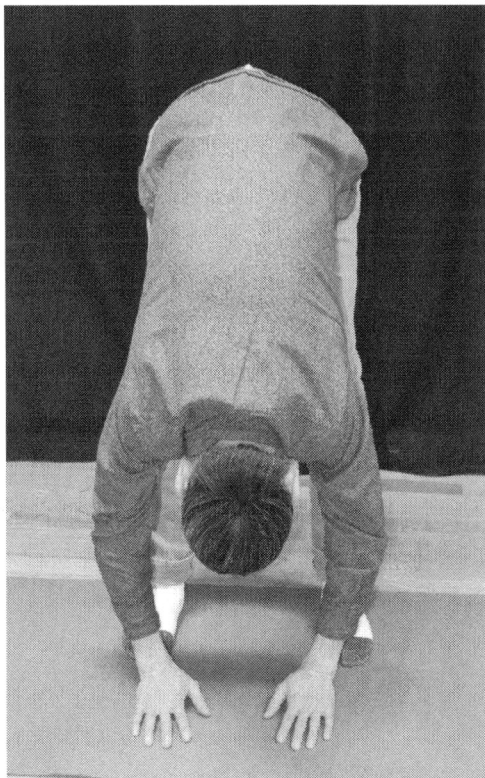

6. Sitting forward bend

This exercise stretches the hamstrings, lower back and tendons behind the knees. As we get older these muscles tighten and become shorter making our legs weaker.

This also contributes to bad posture, which constricts our organs making them less efficient. We become tired more easily and are more susceptible to various health complaints.

- Sit on the floor with your spine erect and your legs close together.

- Reach your arms above your head, and then bending from the hip, reach forward for your feet.

- Try to hold on to your two big toes, sides of feet or the backs of the knees if you are not able to reach your feet. Then gently pull yourself forward.

- Start to take some deep breaths and relax in the pose whilst always reaching forward.

- Hold for one to three minutes and relax.

Sitting forward bend

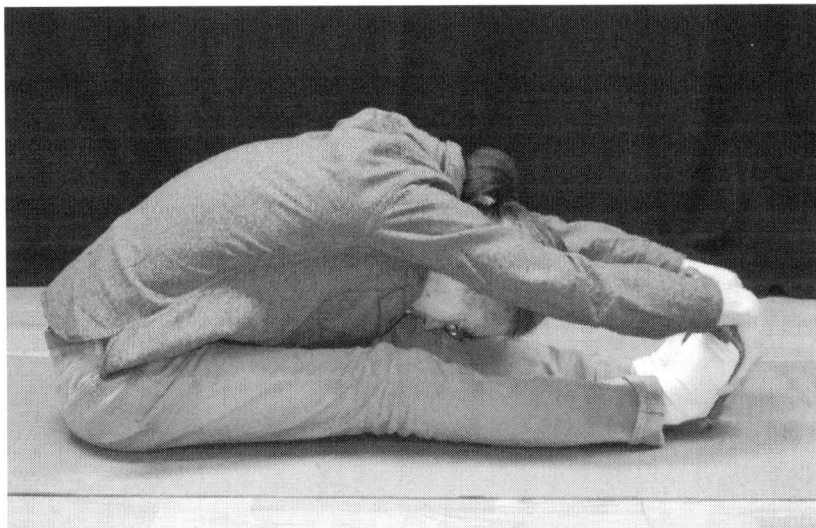

7. Wide leg sitting forward bend pose

This is a variation of the forward bend pose which stretches the inner parts of the leg more.

- Sit on the floor with legs stretched in front of you and your spine erect.

- Open your legs as wide as they can go.

- Breathe in and reach your arms to the sky. As you breathe out, reach forward and touch the floor in front of you.

- Keep reaching your arms in front of your body. Over time, you will be able to touch your chest on the floor.

- Hold for one minute and release. If you want to vary the stretch, you can alternatively try to touch your left foot with your hands for thirty seconds and then your right foot to stretch the sides of the body.

Wide leg sitting forward bend pose

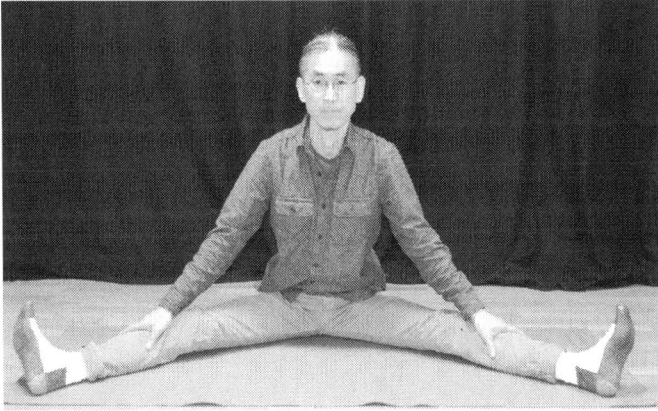

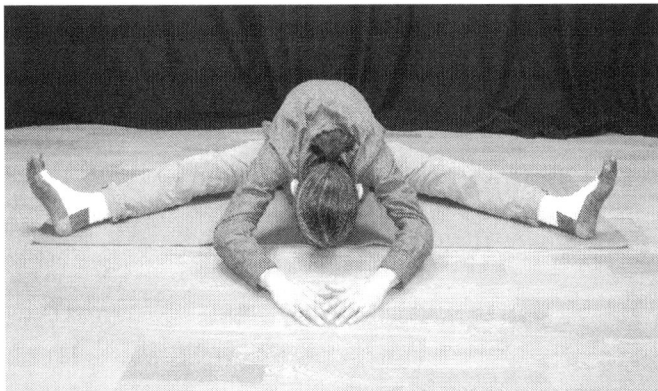

Some people practice the Asian arts of yoga, tai chi or qigong every morning to achieve the same effect on the body. However, these practices are not everybody's cup of tea. These simple exercises in this section break down some of the more essential activities and can be carried out in short periods of time.

The important thing is to do them daily. Tight muscles can over time become shortened and lead to poor circulation, aches and pains. Gently opening up our bodies regularly can help prevent this.

CHAPTER SIX

QIGONG

Qigong / Ki-Ko

Qigong is a series of physical postures, movements practiced with intention and breathing exercises designed to encourage a smooth flow of Qi/Ki energy in the body. The term 'Ki-Ko', is the Japanese name for Qigong.

Exercises may involve gentle movements particularly using the arms or static postures. There are many variations of exercises designed to activate and smooth the flow of Qi/Ki in specific Channel pathways or to simply build up the Qi/Ki energy of the body.

The Chinese word 'Qi' refers to energy. 'Gong' means accomplishment, skill or simply work. Qigong can be practiced for the development of martial arts, medical or for spiritual development. There are hard and soft forms of Qigong. The harder forms are used in martial arts. The softer forms more for health promotion.

There are a great many health benefits to developing a daily practice of qigong. However, like anything in life, it can be abused or overused and result in harmful effects on the body if practiced excessively or in the wrong way. It is best to seek a good teacher or attend a class for guidance.

Some people, particularly the very young become excited when they first start learning qigong and are seduced by expectations of esoteric experiences or developing supernatural power. However excess practice, particularly that which is driven from ego can result in disturbances in your Ki/Qi flow and potentially upset your general mental health.

There are a great many books on the subject with exercises which are worth doing. However, here we will look at the most basic and the most fundamental exercise: 'Holding the Balloon'.

Qigong: Holding the Balloon

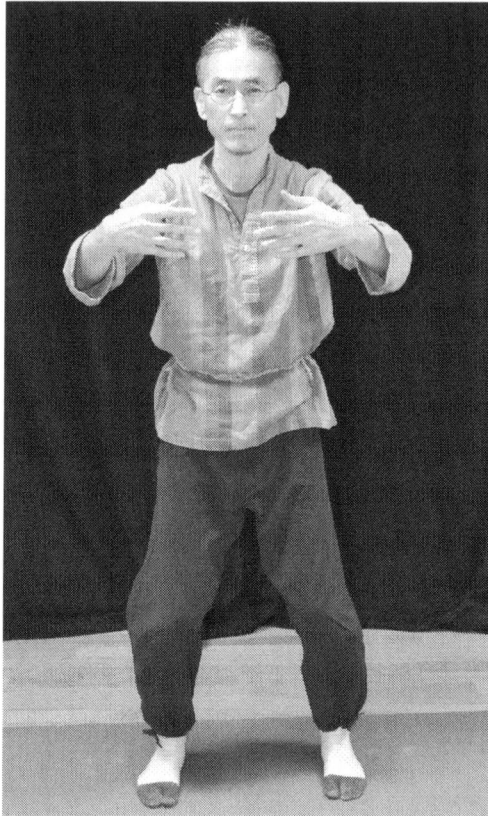

Holding the Balloon Exercise

- Place your feet shoulder-width apart, with feet facing forward.

- Bend the knees slightly. Sink into your hips.

- Keep your back straight and slightly lean forward.

- Imagine your chin being drawn towards the back of your neck.

- Imagine you are holding invisible tennis balls under both of your armpits. Hold your arms in front of your chest and imagine you are holding an invisible balloon in front of your body.

- Keep your eyes slightly closed and breathe through your nose.

- Hold the pose for 5 minutes.

Holding the Balloon

Though it looks like you are simply standing, it is deceptively difficult. If you are not used to the pose, you may find your legs trembling and becoming very tired. You may even sweat. Some more advanced practitioners will hold the pose for up to an hour each time they practice, but building up to doing it for 20 minutes is plenty.

This pose draws Ki energy into your energy centre and allows Ki to circulate throughout your body. An advanced pose is where you lower your stance. Some people can go as low as keeping the tops of their thighs parallel to the ground. This low pose is not necessary for health benefits but from a fitness perspective, it will greatly strengthen your legs.

Though I have described the pose, it is far better to attend a class so the teacher can correct your posture and make sure you are in the correct form. There are also various Qigong exercises, the most famous being the Eight Pieces of Brocade, which are eight basic exercises.

The benefit of Qigong as compared to going to the gym is that most people can easily and safely practice these exercises regardless of age and their health condition. They are versatile and can be carried out at home or in hotel rooms. Also, many of the exercises can be modified. For example, if you are unable to stand, many of the exercises can be carried out seated.

There is also a large body of scientific research into the benefits of qigong particularly on the immune system.

Qigong modulates the immune system

In one study   - 'Qigong: Assessment of Immunological Parameters following a Qigong Training Program', the effects of daily qigong on the immune system was researched. (Manzaneque et al 2004)

The study was carried out at the University of Malaga in Spain. 29 subjects were assessed with 16 of them practicing daily qigong and the rest acting as a control group. The experimental subjects underwent a daily qigong practice of 30 minutes for one month, practicing the set of Qigong exercises called the Eight Pieces of Brocade. These are 8 simple exercises consisting of gentle movements with breathing.

The day before the experiment and one day after its finish, blood samples were taken to record the levels of immunological parameters (leucocytes, immunoglobulins and complement). After 30 days of Qigong practice the exercise group was found to have lower numbers of total leucocytes, eosinophils, monocytes and complement C3 concentrations compared to the control group.

What this showed is that daily Qigong practice has significant effects on the immune system. Though it seems that lower levels of immune cell makers may seem a negative thing, actually it indicated that qigong practice had an effect on modulating the immune system - particularly one that is overactive (as shown in many autoimmune diseases).

For example, C3 factors are known to be markers of inflammation in the body and high levels is said to be associated with pathological conditions including atherosclerotic processes. High levels of monocytes are also associated with inflammatory bowel conditions such as Crohn's disease and rheumatoid arthritis. Likewise, high levels of eosinophils are also seen in asthma and allergic rhinitis and high levels of neutrophils are associated with stress.

This study may well show that Qigong can help with the problem of an overactive immune system and may be beneficial in chronic diseases of the immune system.

Qigong improves quality of life scores in cancer patients

In another study – 'Impact of Medical Qigong on quality of life, fatigue, mood and inflammation in cancer patients (Oh et al 2009)', the effects of qigong in cancer sufferers was researched.

162 adult patients diagnosed with any type of cancer and with an expected survival length of over 12 months were recruited for a trial where they would undergo two 90 minutes sessions of qigong a week for 10 weeks.

The sessions involved 30-minute gentle stretching and typical standing qigong movements to stimulate the bodies channels as well as 15 minutes of exercise in seated positions and 30 minutes of meditating and breathing exercises. They were encouraged to practice at home. The participants were assessed for levels of quality of life, fatigue, mood and an inflammatory biomarker (C-reactive protein (CRP) at the beginning and after 10 weeks of the trial.

After 10 weeks, it was found that participants who practiced Qigong had notable improvements in their quality of life scores, they had significant improvements in their fatigue levels and a greater reduction in mood disturbances and there were again effects on the immune system with differences in the level of the inflammatory biomarker.

The only non-improvement was that there was no difference between the qigong group and the control group in their level of anger, hostility and confusion.

For a very gentle type of exercise, qigong very clearly brings positive changes to the body and has an effect on modulating the immune system.

Moving people with Ki-energy

There are other curious things about the art of Qigong. In London, I was fortunate to regularly attend a qigong class taught by a Japanese teacher called Mr. Kurihara. He used the Japanese term 'Ki-Ko' - the Japanese translation of the word qigong meaning Ki-energy Work'.

As a teacher with a background in Karate and Aikido, Mr. Kurihara taught a more dynamic form of Ki-Ko. His exercises included a stronger stretching of the arm and neck muscles to really open up the Channel pathways. He also included challenging variations of the standing poses, which had the potential to be used in Aikido.

In some of his classes he would demonstrate how he could perform aikido throws using Ki energy instead of the use of physical force or utilizing the opponents own momentum. The finale of his class was a kind of Ki-energy transfer exercise whereby each class member would take it in turns to face Mr Kurihara and do a kind of gentle circular pushing and pulling exercise together with touching forearms using very light pressure against each other.

Pushed away with Ki-energy

After pushing and pulling with feet firmly on the ground, suddenly you would feel a great pressure and find yourself being thrown down the hall. Behind you, there would be 'catchers' - other classmates holding cushions to make sure you didn't get thrown too far and end up in the wall.

This was not a physical sensation. Mr. Kurihara was not physically pushing you using force, it was almost like a flood of energy would explode in front of you and you would feel pushed. In fact, the harder you resist against the sensation, the stronger you would get pushed away.

To demonstrate that this was not due to physical force, he would often get you to repeat the pushing and pulling motion with your arms a few inches apart and without any actual physical touch with him, and yet, you would still feel the same pressure and be pushed away down the hall.

On one occasion, I brought a more skeptical friend along to a class. Despite being thrown himself, he looked for a rational reason for how it happened. He felt that Mr Kurihara may have been pushing him away by somehow throwing him off balance. A reasonable assumption - however, this argument not could explain how you are pushed away without actually being in physical contact with him or explain the intensity at which some members could find themselves thrown away.

Even if this was some kind of suggestion, it is very hard to fake being pushed away without it actually looking fake. Not unless you are a good actor. The strength at which a person would be thrown also varied from person to person.

One of the older Japanese ladies would be sent gently fluttering down the room with her arms flapping gently like a butterfly and she would giggle like a young child. Myself and another young lady who were both slim and relatively flexible would be thrown quickly down the hall so much so that I always needed a catcher to stop me flying into the wall. Some of the more stiffer members tended not to be pushed so well despite several attempts.

This ease of movement may well have been an indication of how open the channels were in each person. This exercise always raised lots of laughs and exclamations and demonstrated simply that Ki-energy has the power to be transferred from one to another and can move people. Although, I imagine a lot of people will find this hard to believe until they experience this or something similar for themselves.

Qigong and Tai Chi for Arthritis

When I see a patient, who suffers from arthritis or any kind of muscular pain, I often advise them to seek out a Qigong class or Tai Chi class (a close relation to qigong).

The slow gentle exercises of qigong have a focus on opening up the joints (a common site of arthritis), These exercises also slowly build up strength and endurance. I think that if a person underwent a combination of regular qigong practice along with acupuncture and moxibustion, they may gain many improvements to their mobility and muscular flexibility.

I met two ladies in their 70s who were able to overcome chronic arthritis with regular Tai Chi practice. One of them was a German lady called Dorothea who was my Tai Chi and Qigong teacher in London and who studied under the well-known Sufi teacher Mrs. Irina Tweedie.

Another lady I met was a Chinese woman who was very friendly to me whilst attending a few Micheal Tse classes (a well-known Wing Chun teacher and Tai Chi teacher). My one memory of this lady was watching her holding a spear and leaping through the air as she performed a jumping movement... not bad for a 70-year-old.

頭寒足熱

Zukan Sokunetsu

Keep a cool head and warm feet

Another variation is: '

For health - fire below, water above and a cool head'.

This expression – 'keep a cool head and warm feet', relates to balancing the yin and yang energies of the body.

Activity is yang in nature, with qualities of warmness and heat. Rest and quietness is yin in nature, with qualities of coolness and cold. Modern Western society tends towards excess activity (yang) with the overuse of the brain and sense organs particularly the eyes and ears.

We overuse our eyes and stimulate our brains with computer work, watching TV, surfing the net or browsing our smartphones. We also think or worry too much and are slaves to our desires or stresses. All of this brings energy and heat to the top parts of our body - our brains and eyes creating a Yin Yang imbalance.

Basically, our heads become warmer (yang) and the lower parts of our body become cooler (yin). In some traditions of meditation, it is believed you can cure sickness by meditating on the feet to bring the yang energy down.

In other traditions, meditating is carried out with a focus on the Tantien (the power center of the body), an area in the lower abdomen, which has the effect of drawing down excess yang energy from the top part of the body to the lower part of the body.

In the above phrase 'fire below, water above...', the "water above" relates to the 'heart energy centre'. This also corresponds to the Heart Chakra – a term used in Traditional Indian philosophy referring to one of the seven centres of spiritual power in the human body. The Heart Energy Centre should be calm and not agitated by fire (such as excessive desires or worries). A cool head means we should have a calm head without too much brain activity or thoughts.

A traditional Chinese exercise is to meditate on the lower Tantien area because where the mind goes, the energy follows. If our mind is focused heavily in our brains, the energy flows upwards, but if our minds are focused in our lower belly, the energy flows there and helps keep our energies centered. Another variation, is that we should keep fire in our feet (below) either by meditating on our feet or by regular walking, which brings excess yang energy downwards.

The Tantien (*dantien* in Chinese) is an important area in the lower abdomen. It is approximately two finger-breaths below the bellybutton and is considered to be the main power center of the body.

In a healthy person, the lower belly should be warm, soft and pliant. Any signs of coldness, tightness or hardness in the lower abdomen can be a sign of blockage and is one of the reasons why abdominal palpation is used as a diagnostic tool in Japanese acupuncture and shiatsu.

Traditional Oriental medicine believes that our center and the lower parts of the body need to be warmer. Our lower belly – our Tantien, also houses many important organs such as our kidneys, our intestines, bladder, stomach and liver, which carry out the important work of processing the foods we eat and filtering and removing the wastes in our body.

This activity requires yang energy. If there is not enough yang energy in this part of the body and any of these organs fail to carry out their functions, wastes can build up in the body and make us sick.

This is one of the benefits to practicing deep breathing which brings our energy down to the center and away from our heads as well as avoiding excess stimulation such as computers, TV or Smartphones, especially in the evening when we need to be slowing down ready for sleep.

In the modern age and in certain jobs, excessive brain work or work using the eyes is unavoidable particularly with the many kinds of administrative or computer based jobs these days. For these people, it is essential to balance this excess eye/brain yang work with some kind of practice that doesn't use the brain too much and which instead emphasizes using the full body such as swimming, gardening or yoga.

Or even simply sitting quietly in a meditative pose for 10 or 20 minutes in a quiet dark place particularly at the end of the evening with no outside distractions can help.

The consequence of having a warm head and cold feet are not immediate but can lead to premature ageing and can possibly manifest with some of these signs: - shallow breathing patterns, headaches, unsound sleep, frequent bad dreams, anxiety, a propensity to get overworked or over-stressed more easily, irritability with others, skin eruptions, poor digestive function, IBS type symptoms, feeling cold and frequent urination.

CHAPTER SEVEN

DAILY CHORES AS EXERCISE

A hundred years ago, a person would have no need to go to the gym. Work was more physical and they used their bodies more. On the contrary, it was resting and sitting that would have been useful to them.

Today, our jobs and lives have become more sedentary and we need to counteract this by purposely doing exercise. It is common for people to go to the gym or partake in sports or exercise classes each week in order to maintain a good bodily condition. This is a necessary action today.

However, there are still a great many physical activities we need to carry out today as part of daily life and despite the many attempts of the Japanese to build human-like robots to be our slaves and do all our work for us, their attempts are more akin to Johnny-5 models in 'Short Circuit' or else Lolita-esque pleasure dolls. Neither of which could probably wash the dishes.

The beneficial effects of housework

Housework is by far one of the best forms of daily activity available to us. One example of the benefits of housework can be found in an account of George Ohsawa.

George Ohsawa (1893-1966) is regarded as the founder of Macrobiotics - a popular diet and lifestyle practice that has spread around the world. Macrobiotics is a healthy living eating plan, which recommends a simple Japanese diet based on brown rice, miso soup, Japanese vegetables and condiments and cooking methods. It is a diet that is naturally low in fat, sugar and meat and which claims to confer several health benefits. George Ohsawa was a man of great energy and passion for his movement. He was described as:

> "A person of great, almost boundless physical and mental energy. Even as a man of seventy he walked with a spring in his step and normally bounded up steps two or three at a time. When he walked in the streets, his fast pace would usually leave companions behind."

However, Ohsawa did very little sports. He preferred exercise that was a part of everyday life particularly housework:

> "Ohsawa took particular delight in cleaning, dusting and mopping with a vigor that gave him a good daily workout. As a result of this activity and his generally spartan diet of rice and vegetable, Ohsawa was lean and strong. Once he did a few sessions of judo at a dojo. The teacher, impressed with his leg and lower body strength, asked him how long he had been practicing the martial arts. "Only since I have been coming here" was the reply".

Another example of Ohsawa's enthusiasm for housework and for order and cleanliness was practiced when he travelled:

> "Whenever he stayed as a guest somewhere he would get up early and clean the whole house. While staying at Mme Riviere's Paris apartment in 1961, Ohsawa cleaned the bathroom, and especially a wooden toilet top, with such care, that his hostess thought it was a newly bought fixture. When in 1946, Ohsawa lodged in the Kobayashi house his aim, he said, was not only to maintain the place, but to leave it much improved".

Ohsawa's example of his enthusiasm for housework is a little extreme and reflected his strict and disciplined nature, which may have been peculiar to his samurai heritage and upbringing in a harder world. Nonetheless, the act of keeping the room clean with regular housework also ensures a smooth flow of energy in your living environment.

Dirt and clutter stagnates and can breed negative feelings in whoever lives in this house. This is *feng shui* at its most basic - the art of spatially arranging objects, furniture, structures or buildings in a way to harmonize the flow of energy around you.

Minimalism

It is hard to adequately define what Minimalism is as there are many interpretations. I would define minimalism as the following of a simpler life, the removal of distractions and focusing on the most important things to your life.

It may be the practice of downscaling your life, living with fewer possessions such as not owning a car or television, foregoing holidays or too many clothes and removing things around you that are distracting you from your purpose in life.

The concept of Minimalism has grown in popularity in Japan and has been paired with the Zen Buddhism philosophy of the 'simplicity of life' to influence the Japanese into adopting minimalist home environments.

> "The process is more than de-cluttering, but re-evaluating what possessions mean, to gain something else more important", (Lim 2016).

It seems a relevant concept in a world where the accumulation of goods, particularly as a reflection of status and waste have become trademarks of our society. It may be that these times will pass and we may have to return to a time of thrift and valuing what we do have again in the future.

Another principle of minimalism is quality. Today it is possible to buy a large set of cheap cups and cutlery, mass produced in China by workers in near slave-like conditions. Or we can buy low cost garments in our high street shops made in factory workshops in India, Bangladesh or Vietnam in some cases made by children. Or flat screen TVs, and any number of electronics such as bread makers, coffee machines or toasters.

We collect CDs and DVDs. Makeup is cheap and some women have boxes full of it. But for the most part, we do not really appreciate it because there is no true love in the making of any of it.

The concept of Japanese minimalism is to only buy one or two top quality items of clothes, shoes or makeup and use them. Because it is of higher quality and more expensive, it can last many years and we will be more inclined to look after it, keeping it clean, repairing it and generally appreciating it more.

This is one of the reasons why vintage fashion is so popular. How can a dress made in the 1960's cost more than a dress made this year?

The reason is that it was produced to a higher standard. The material is of a higher quality, it will have been produced in England by people with normal lives, not by women in slave-like conditions in China. It will also have been cared for over many years so that even 50 years later, it is still as desirable as when it was first made. I can't imagine many high street shop clothes still being sold 50 years in the future. Some of them don't even last one year.

Shopping, buying and collecting things can reflect an underlying sign of stress and unhappiness in your life. Some people will frequently go shopping and buy many items of clothing even though they may never wear them. Some people buy many clothes on credit slowly accumulating debt.

The collecting of objects only compounds the problems, because as the house becomes more cluttered, it clouds the mind making the person less focused mentally and spiritually.

The best action is to clear out the house, sell off what is not needed or give it away. Clean and reduce what you need to just a few high-quality items that you use often. With the exception of a suit, which everyone needs for special occasions - weddings, christenings, funerals, meetings or interviews, if something is sitting in your cupboard that you never wear but that you are saving for *the right time*, which hasn't happened yet, then just get rid of it.

As you clear clutter, your mind becomes clearer. You can only invite new positive experiences, people and higher quality objects into your life by first removing the clutter and stagnations.

Gardening

If we look at images of Japanese Zen gardens, we see works of art in a landscape form. Every plant, pebble and tree is shaped and arranged with an incredible precision. These plants are maintained on a daily basis as a labour of love and gives us an example of how beauty and art can be fashioned from even something as simple as a garden.

Gardens are a place for us to relax in during sunny days or to play in for children. There can be a sense of pride in maintaining a garden and keeping a tidy front lawn. If you have an allotment or grow vegetables, then you have the opportunity to save money on vegetables and also to work your bodies as there are always weeds to pull up, beds to maintain, mulch to spread, shrubs and trees to cut back, bulbs to plant, fences to repair, and seeds to prepare.

Gardening work is another activity that can keep us fit and healthy as it requires us to use all our muscles in digging, bending over, planting out, watering, cutting grass and trimming hedges.

Also, the exposure to the daylight sun helps our body obtain vitamin D, which is good for our bone health. My father, now in his late 70s still regularly grows and eats his own vegetables and I would attribute his longevity due to his regular gardening work and consumption of his own natural, organically grown vegetables.

For millennia, humans have had a close relationship to the soil. The food we grow in the ground keeps us alive and nourishes us. However, as urban living becomes more common, it is easy to forget that those green vegetables bought in the supermarket wrapped up in colourful labelled packets actually came from the ground.

Gardening also puts us in close proximity to plenty of oxygen spewing plants which can have a calming effect on us and reduce our stress levels.

CHAPTER EIGHT

DEEP BREATHING

Aside from meditation, deep breathing is one of the most effective ways to deal with stress. During an acupuncture treatment, I often observe that once the needles have been inserted, a person's breathing pattern changes. Their breathing may become longer and deeper. The lower abdomen expands quite noticeably and it feels almost like a release of tension has occurred.

The same can occur during a massage treatment, or even after talking with a client and allowing them to talk and offload some stress or pent up emotions, their breathing pattern may become more relaxed and deeper.

As you breathe deeply, the lungs expand and the diaphragm - the muscle responsible for breathing, pushes further downwards, which in turn massages the internal organs - the liver, kidney, intestines and also the heart above. This *internal* massage helps encourage a smooth flow of Ki energy and circulation within the internal organs.

The diaphragm functions in breathing

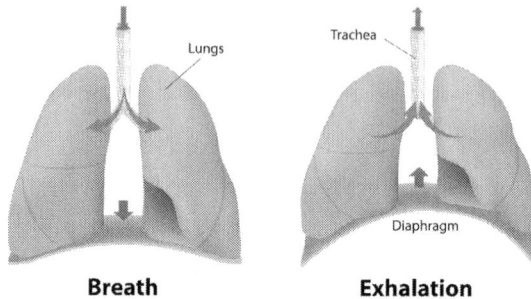

Breath   **Exhalation**

In this diagram, on the left, deep breathing expands all three lobes of the lung, pushing the diaphragm muscle downwards, which in turns massages all the internal organs below - the intestines, kidneys and liver.

Many people have shallow breathing patterns. Shallow breathing means that we are using a small percentage of our lung capacity to breathe in and out and that we have less fresh oxygen flowing into the body and less waste being removed. It means that in the lower lobes of their lungs there will be more stale air.

If we really want to optimize our health, we should learn to gradually breathe deeper and fuller and utilize more of our lung power. Just take a moment and observe your own breathing right now without trying to change anything and take note. Is it shallow? Are you breathing more into your upper chest? Are your breaths hurried and short?

Stress changes our breathing patterns. It makes us breathe shorter and quicker and mostly in the upper part of our lungs. If we are regularly affected by stressful situations in our everyday life, a quick and shallow breathing pattern becomes almost fixed and will affect our personality accordingly.

When we consciously take a few deep breaths, almost immediately we can feel calmer. In Chinese medicine, The Lungs govern Ki. They take in Ki from the universe. The more deeper and calmer we breathe, the more Ki we take in and the more Ki is able to flow in our bodies. This can lead us to feel calmer and healthier. If we were to practice breathing exercise for ten minutes when we wake up and ten minutes before we go to bed, we can start to create a different breathing pattern.

In Japan, Toru Abo was a well-known Professor, Medical doctor and professor at the Department of Immunology School of Medicine in Niigata University who had gained an international reputation for his research on immune cells. He is also famous for advocating natural approaches and therapies in the treatment of diseases such as cancer.

His outspoken criticism of the standard medical approach to cancer – chemotherapy, surgery and radiotherapy earned him a controversial reputation.

In his book 'The Only Two Causes of All Diseases', Toru talks about the importance of the mitochondrial pathway and that when people are not adequately using this pathway, cancer and other diseases are a risk.

His hypothesis is that a continuous bodily environment of lack of oxygen in the body's tissues (hypoxia) along with an abnormal low-body temperature (hypothermia) as well as an over-dependency on the glycolysis pathway (the system that converts nutrients from food into energy) instead of the mitochondrial pathway (where nutrients are produced from both food and energy from breathing) are factors that can put the body at risk of cancer.

Toru advises:

> 'It is very important to inhale a lot of oxygen into your body by practicing deep breathing. When you get sick, you would breathe heavily, which shows that the body is requiring you to breathe in more because your body is in a state of hypoxia (a condition in which the body or part is deprived of sufficient oxygen).
>
> Same thing can be said when you get angry or irritated, your breath becomes shallow or you may hold your breath. If the irritating situation continues, then the hypoxia becomes chronic. With shallow breathing, obviously not all body cells are getting enough oxygen".

Simple Breathing Exercise

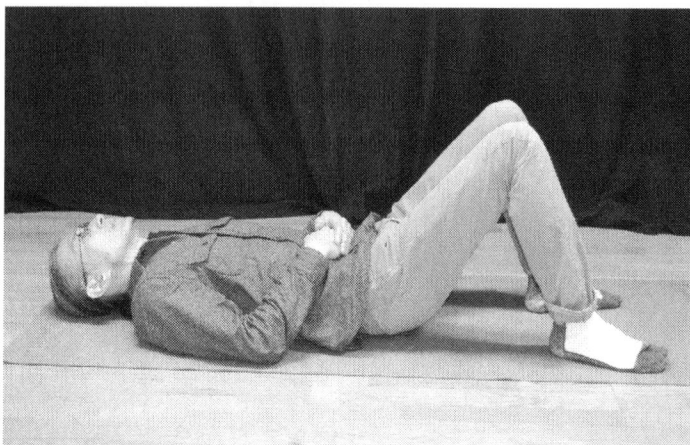

Lie on your back on a comfortable mat on the floor. Let your muscles relax into the floor. Place your hands on your lower belly (hara), one on top of the other. Relax in this pose.

Breathe in through your nose with long and slow breaths into your lower belly. As you breathe in, feel your hara expand outwards. Breathe out slowly and gently. As you breathe out, feel your hara sink back in. Take 10 more breaths like this, feeling your hara expand and sink back in again. After you have taken your ten deep breaths, relax in the pose and be aware of how your body feels.

I have practiced this type of breathing with groups of people including healthcare professionals, carers and the elderly. Though the majority will feel immediately calmer and sometimes even more reflective or contemplative after practicing this breathing, there may be someone who feels a little lightheaded or finds the exercise uncomfortable.

Some people are so used to breathing shallowly in the upper chest or have had so much stress to deal with in their lives, that shallow breathing has become a part of their normal body pattern. When they then suddenly practice deep breathing, they may find themselves feeling lightheaded, dizzy or even have headaches. If you feel this happen to you, stop the exercise and just relax.

Perhaps slowly build up the exercise by taking one or two deep breaths every now and again until your body gets used to it is a more cautious approach. There is nothing inherently bad in taking deep breaths but if your body is not used to it, it can be too much, too soon and a shock to the system. It may not be suitable for some people who suffer from lung diseases such as COPD or Lung cancer as their breathing is already problematic.

This exercise can be practiced sitting in seiza or a cross-legged position. Or on a straight back chair sitting upright. In fact, it can be utilized at any time of the day and is particularly useful when we find ourselves under a sudden stressful situation requiring quick decisions and we want to maintain a calm mind in order to deal with the problem.

Qigong Deep Breathing Exercises for Health

Geoff Pike (born 1929) was a British born naturalised Australian with a variety of life experiences. He worked as a deck boy in the British navy during the Second World War. He was a soldier, lumberjack, a cartoonist and a successful advertising executive.

Whilst living in Hong Kong, he had the revelation, that although he was successful and enjoying the *good life*, his physical health was in a poor state. Soon after, he was introduced to the health preservation exercise of qigong and in particular the deep breathing exercises, which he started diligently practicing.

Unfortunately, in 1977 he was diagnosed with throat cancer. Instead of only following the conventional medical approach to cancer, Geoff used his Qigong breathing exercises at first to help him deal with the side effects of radiotherapy and then continued to treat himself using his deep breathing exercises. He healed his cancer and still 30 years later, he was still alive and writing books under his adopted name of Pai Kit Fai. His long life was a testimony to the potential power of qigong.

On breathing, the Qigong master Geoff Pike attributed deep breathing exercises to being able to heal his own cancer. In his book: The Power of Qi, he discusses how poor breathing habits are very common and that regular breathing exercises can potentially increase your lung capacity and the size of your chest:

"The percentage of civilized men who breathe correctly is quite small, and the result is shown in contracted chests and stooping shoulders, and the terrible increase in diseases of the respiratory organs.

Begin practicing deep breathing whenever and wherever it occurs to you to do so, while walking, resting, working or even preparing for sleep. Make regular, conscious efforts to increase your breath load. during this process, your ribcage will expand and with it, the ease and capacity of your respiration. You may find that you gain up to 2 cm around the chest. In a month's time, it may have expanded another 2 cm or even more to the full extent your frame will allow…"

When I trained for my acupuncture license over 10 years ago, one of my class mates was a strongly-built man called Glen. Glen had undergone many years of training in Qigong and in particular the qigong breathing exercises. As a result, he had a loud booming voice and a strong charismatic presence. As an Irishman, he also liked to enjoy a drink and had no restrictions with his diet as he told me, his hard training meant he could digest anything.

As one of my assignments, he taught me a special breathing exercise that he had been practicing for years and confided in me that in the past, he had been very thin but it was from the years of breathing exercises, that he had built his strength and size.

CHAPTER NINE

STRESS AND TENSION AND ITS EFFECT ON HEALTH AND DISEASE

Daily life has many stresses that we must deal with as part of the human experience. Financial problems, workplace stresses, relationships, commuting are some of them. Even our entertainment and media such as the daily news brings stresses.

Stress is not a modern invention. Our ancestors have been dealing with it for centuries. In fact, they probably had it worse. Imagine your daily stress was whether you would be able to feed your family through the winter. The ancient Chinese had their share of problems. They too would have been affected by food shortages, money, work problems, marital disharmony and sickness.

Stress has always been a part of life. It is probably in the modern period that we have given it a label. Stress causes many problems. Apart from the constant feeling of anxiety, uncertainty and worry that accompanies it, if it is severe, it can lead to insomnia, loss of appetite, overeating, digestive problems, headaches and gynecological problems.

In relationships, it can lead to more arguments between family members. It can lead to self-destructive behavior like over-drinking, smoking too much, drug use (both illicit or prescription) or general irritability towards others. Or it can turn inwards leading to depression and potentially lead to suicidal thoughts.

Stress is an important part of life and in some situations, it can be positive. The human body is designed to deal with stress. It keeps the body alert and able to avoid danger. Unfortunately, modern day living can be stressful in a peculiarly negative way.

The scientist Hans Selye showed the negative effects of stress with his model called the General Adaptive Syndrome (GAS). In his work, he subjected laboratory rats to stress (by torturing them). Unsurprisingly, many of them became very sick, suffering intestinal ulcers, wasting away of the thymus and enlargement of the adrenal glands.

In his theory of the general adaptive syndrome (GAS), the body goes through three stages when dealing with stress: Alarm, Resistance and Recovery or Exhaustion. In the 'alarm' stage, stress appears.

For example, when a boss is always pressuring us in the workplace we have to grit our teeth and suppress our feelings for 40 hours a week. Or if we are verbally or mentally bullied by a spouse over a long period of time. Or when a final reminder for a bill comes in and we can't afford to pay it causing us sleepless nights.

All these situations create the stress response which unfortunately cannot be dealt with immediately. Instead we must suppress our natural stress reaction and in some cases, the stress response continues to affect us past the resistance stage and into the exhaustion stage possibly even leading us to develop illnesses which don't always get attributed to stress but perhaps should be.

The long-term effects of stress begin to drain the body causing wear and tear. This can cause headaches, stomach ulcers, constipation, cardiovascular disease, depression, anxiety and sleep problems. Stress also inhibits digestion causing weight gain and depletes the body of many vitamins and minerals necessary for healthy function. Many people use tobacco or alcohol to relieve the stress but these do not get at the root cause.

The worse effects are on the immune system. The immune system produces white blood cells: T-lymphocytes that protect the body from bacteria, infections and cancer cells. High levels of stress suppress these T-lymphocytes, which weakens the immune system and makes the body more vulnerable to infections and colds. We take longer to recover from them and experience much worse symptoms.

Another type of stress that is very typical of the modern world is the stress of overwork. Many jobs place huge demands on people. Today people are expected to do the same work that two or three people would have done twenty or thirty years ago. There is more pressure of deadlines, targets and far less job security.

The general trend is that employees are squeezed more and paid less. Coupled with this are inflation rates that are higher than officially stated by governments resulting in financial stresses for many families.

All of these factors create a kind of artificial stress that is actually more harmful. The reason is that this stress is constant and it also impacts on all areas of people's lives.

In Japan, there is a word karoshi. It literally means '*death by overwork*' and was coined after several Japanese salarymen died prematurely from working an excess of hours, not taking holidays, lacking sleep or working when very sick. Work stress is especially pernicious. It is not just the worker being affected. It also affects their family, their marriage and relationships. Ultimately it impacts the community and society as a whole if our productive members are being killed off prematurely.

People who are stressed and tired at work invariably take this stress home with them, where it affects the family and can leads to disharmonious family relationships. It may create a cycle of stress at home, which then gets passed on to other family members, including children who take this stress to school where they play-up more, become withdrawn or bully others, which in turn passes on stress to their teachers or other students.

If any other stressful situation is added to the mix such as a loss of job or income, a problem with a family member, sickness or bereavement, it all provides a further drain to our bodies and immune system. It may even be a contributory factor to the increasing rates of chronic diseases and cancer in the Western world in the last 70 years.

Exercise and Stress

As too much *bad* stress makes us sick and tired. One way to counteract this is to cool down the *fight or flight* response and give the body what it needs. The body is prepared for physical activity, so that's exactly what we should do. If we do vigorous exercise to the point of sweating, we metabolize excess stress hormones and also release endorphins – hormones that lift the mood and make us physically and mentally calmer.

There are various ways to do this. If we are stressed, exercise, sports, running, swimming or calisthenics can help metabolize these excess stress hormones. Or long walks at a fast pace can help. The worse reaction is sitting down and brooding in a pit of darkness on the problem.

Yang Lifestyles and the Hurry-up West

A very common source of stress and tension in the modern world is that of over-stimulation. In traditional Chinese medicine this refers to an excess of 'joy'. It may seem strange that an excess of joy can be a cause of illness, but I think a good example can be found in Leonardo DiCaprio's portrayal of the corrupt and hard-living stockbroker Jordan Belfort in the movie 'The Wolf of Wall Street'.

Jordan is a loud, overly confident man addicted to drugs, sex and making money. He is successful and seemingly unstoppable. However, he goes too far and eventually his life falls to pieces and he ends up in prison.

In this movie, we see an extreme version of how 'joy' can lead to disharmony. It is simply an extreme example of the Yang orientated nature of modern Western life, which favors overstimulation, growth and over-activity.

腹も身の内

Hara mo minouchi

'Moderation is its own medicine'

This Japanese proverb – 'moderation is its own medicine', can refer to many things - to diet, to sex, to work, to play. It can also refer to activity. We need to be aware of when we are pushing ourselves or doing too much and to balance the Yin and Yang of our bodies.

CHAPTER TEN

TENSION AND THE FASCIA LAYER

Stress = Tension

The word 'stress' evolved from the Latin word 'strictus', which means 'tight, compressed or to draw together'. If we consider the meaning of these words, we can see that stress can be interpreted as a compression and tightness of the body, resulting in a hindered flow of Ki energy in the body.

This tightness, which I also refer to as 'tension' can impair health by restricting the Ki-energy flow to the internal organs resulting in overactive or underactive organ functioning as well as through the muscles leading to muscular pain. If this 'tension' is particularly severe or it continues a long time, then the impact on our health is more significant.

As we mentioned, the word "stress" comes from the Latin "strictus", meaning 'drawn tight'. In relation to the human body, this is exactly what stress does to the body. It draws us in tight. It creates tension in our musculature, our skin, our fascia, even our organs. When someone is stressed, typically they frown or clench their jaws or their fists. They draw themselves tight.

If stress is continuous, these kinds of physical reactions can lead to wrinkles or frown lines on the face. Maybe they find themselves involuntarily grinding their teeth in their sleep. Perhaps after 20 or thirty years, they develop arthritis in those hands that have been clenched so much. These are visible signs of tension, but the effects of tension are systemic and affect the whole body.

Stress equates to tension. Tension restricts Ki-energy flow. Poor Ki-energy flow leads to health problems. This is why Oriental medicine and the health practices of tai chi, yoga and qigong can be very beneficial to the body because they release this tension. If we practiced just ten minutes a day of qigong meditative exercise we could perhaps release some of the effects of tension and stress that otherwise could make us sick years in the future.

Sickness is caused by the holding of tension in the 'body energetic'. By the energetic I refer to the body in total – the muscle zones, the fascia, the bones, the joints, the blood and the skin, all of which encompass the Channel pathways and acupuncture points.

Tension is also held as a result of trauma, overuse or misuse of the body, along with prior sickness which has not been completely resolved and has gone deeper into the body. Latent viral infections or 'stuck heat' also fall under this category. Emotional stress also causes tension. For example, strong emotions such as anger, grief, unrealised ambition, resentment, inferiority, unresolved frustrations, even excessive desire can disturb the body energetic.

Working men and women, for example, farmers, manual labourers or gardeners are prone to tensions of the muscular skeletal zones. Modern day people – the educated or 'civilised' are more at risk of emotional-distress tension.

Energy circulates in the body. When the energy flow is disturbed due to tension, Ki-energy stagnates or flows irregularly. Then we see the manifestation of symptoms. Some of these imbalances can be observed in the posture or can be palpated in areas of the body. They may also be reflected in the attitudes, mindset, character and emotions of the person. If someone receives treatment early on such as acupuncture or massage at this time, it may be able to resolve some of the tension.

One of the objectives of an acupuncture treatment may be to release this tension. Other practices such as meditation, healing, and other physical therapies may help to release the body energetic. Some problems may be resolved. Some may not. The ultimate release of body tension is death but we do not want to have to wait for that, so it is better to take steps to achieve release of the body energetic during our lifetimes.

Children are born relatively free of tension, but as they grow older and experience 'life' and all its challenges and some bad habits, they will gradually build up tension in the body energetic by the time they are middle-aged.

Tension is a factor in body disharmony and disease.

If tension builds up, or is unresolved and continues for a long time, it pushes the body beyond its natural ability to handle it and the body becomes weaker. Then there is a potential for it to break down at its weakest part. The weakest part may either be an area that has been strained under an excessive level of tension (for example the liver organ of an alcoholic), or it could be where you have a constitutional weakness.

Humans tend to be born with constitutional organs or parts that are relatively weak and other areas that are relatively strong. Often tension may cause the break-down at the constitutionally weak area of the body. In some cases, there is a trigger that sets off an illness. The proverbial straw that broke the camel's back which may come in the form of a sudden bereavement, accident or stress like a loss of job or divorce.

Tension can be caused by unresolved infections, surgeries, physical, mental or emotional stress, unresolved accidents, incompletely healed injuries, drugs, alcohol abuse, negative moods, mental or physical abuse, bad parenting, bullying, work stress, over-exercise, lack of exercise, over-eating, under-eating, poison, pollution, bereavement or trauma.

Another form of tension in the body actually comes from blockages due to excessive inactivity such as laziness, enforced idleness such as from loss of a job, or types of boredom caused when someone does not have a daily purpose and suffers mildly from depression.

Humans are optimistic organisms, but the reality is that life is full of problems. Sometimes we have no control over problems. However, we do have some control over how we deal with them and we would do well to develop our ability to learn how to deal and handle stresses in life. We must learn to be more resilient.

Fortunately, there are many simple ways to release tension. One of the best things we can do in our daily life is to spend a little time - even just 15 minutes a day to release some of this tension. Your older self will thank you for it.

The fascia layer and plaque

Some acupuncturists believe that the channel system is not so much a series of Channel pathways or meridians which traverse the body but which actually refer to the fascia layers – the connective tissue that covers every muscle and organ in the body. Very little is known about this fascia layer. Certainly, the Channel pathways may traverse the fascia layers and in this way, it would be beneficial to keep the fascia layers free of restriction.

If it is true that the Channel system of acupuncture is actually an analogy of the fascia layer, then a sticky or blocked fascia layer would be inconducive to energy flow and general health. Fortunately, the solution to this is in movement and exercise.

If the body is a canvas reflecting our life experiences, then taking a close look at it in death may reveal a deeper understanding of our health. One such body worker did just that by creating a series of videos based on his dissection work on cadavers. Gill Hedley's, 'Integral Anatomy' courses represent a useful insight into understanding and appreciating the interconnectedness of the body and layers particularly by examining the fascia levels.

His videos are available for free on YouTube and it is worth looking if you are serious about studying any type of bodywork therapy. In one of his videos, he talks about fascia and stretching as he dissects a cadaver. As he separates the fascia layers from the muscle, he encounters a thin white silky plaque-like substance that he calls "fuzz". This is a transcription of his description of this plaque-like substance from one of his videos:

> "The fuzz yields to my fingertips. Sometimes the fuzz doesn't yield to my fingertips. A stronger, thicker strand that doesn't yield to my fingertips that represents older fuzz. But each night when you go to sleep, the interfaces between your muscles grow fuzz, and in the mornings when you wake up and stretch the fuzz melts.
>
> That stiff feeling you have is the solidifying of your tissues, the sliding surfaces aren't sliding anymore. There's fuzz growing in between them, you need to stretch. Every cat in the world gets up in the morning and it stretches its body and it melts the fuzz and the same way that the fuzz melted when I passed my finger through it, when you're moving, it's as though you are passing your finger through the fuzz just like I did on the cadaver".

In this extract, Gill describes a white plaque-type substance that encases the interfaces between the muscles and which stops the muscles from sliding smoothly over each other. In some places, this fuzz easily breaks apart as he passes his hands through them, but in other places it has built up and solidified hindering the sliding surfaces.

Gill explains how this layer can easily be removed with some light movement and gentle exercises such as a simple stretching routine in the morning. However, if this plaque layer is allowed to build up, such as where the person has a very sedentary lifestyle, it hardens and actually leads to restriction in the fascia layer in a similar way that plaque can harden and build up into tarter on the teeth.

This hardened tissue no doubt leads to a restriction of muscle mobility and from a Traditional Oriental Medical point of view, restricts the flow of Ki-energy flow in the body. Gill advises:

> "So you have to stretch and move and use your body in order to melt the fuzz that's building up between the sliding surfaces of your musculature, these sliding surfaces (of the muscles) and this fuzz is all over your body.
>
> Now what happens when you get an injury? My shoulder is stiff now. I'm holding my shoulder. I go to bed. I wake up in the morning. I don't stretch my shoulder. I'm afraid it hurts. Last night's fuzz doesn't get melted away. I go to bed, I sleep some more. Now I have two nights fuzz built up. Now two nights fuzz is more fuzz than one night's fuzz. What if I have a week's fuzz or a month's fuzz?
>
> Now these fuzz fibres start lining up and intertwining and all of a sudden you have thicker fibres forming. You start to have an inhibition of the potential for movement. It's no longer a simple matter of having a stretch. Now you need some work. Now you might need to do a more systematic exploration of that place to restore the original movement that you lost and usually this is the case if you have a temporary injury and then we restore our movement...
>
> The buildup of fuzz amongst the sliding surfaces, our surfaces that our motion becomes limited or limited cycles become introduced into our normal range of movement. We start to walk around like this. We are all fuzzed over. Our body is literally solidifying. We are reducing our natural range of movement in individual areas of the body and in our entire body in general".

Here Gill talks about what happened when this plaque-like substance is not removed but instead it builds up restricting movement between muscles and effectively making us tight. Gill advises:

"I believe that one of the great benefits of bodywork be it massages or any kind of hands on therapies are that they introduce movement manually to tissues that have become fuzzed over through lack of movements whether it is because of an injury and a person is protecting that injury or because of personality expression.

So you can grow fuzz by choice or by accident, but you can take responsibility for melting the fuzz and if there's too much fuzz in your body and it's frozen up, you might want to seek help in order to introduce movement so there, the new cycle has a little more movement and a little more movement instead of a little less movement.

Fuzz represents time. The easiest it is for me to pass my finger through it, the less amount of time it's been there. If I have to use a scalpel to dig my way through one otherwise sliding surface, I know that's been building up for a long time. So you can see time in fuzz."

Traditional Oriental bodywork therapies like acupuncture or massage are some of the interventions that can help to release this fuzz. If the Traditional Chinese Medicine concept of Channel networks did actually refer to the fascia layers, then it is logical to conclude that this fuzz would represent a blockage of the flow of Ki in these Channels, potentially having a negative effect on the health of the body. It could also lead to restrictive movement problems such as arthritis and frozen shoulder.

It is not inconceivable to assume that fuzz building up and solidifying can occur with habitual body holding patterns. For example, a child growing up in an unpleasant household or a long-term depressed person with slumped shoulders may have a build-up of fuzz in the pectoral muscles restricting their breathing and leaving them feeling even more depressed.

Releasing Tension in the Body Energetic

The ultimate release of all body tension, is death. It is the final release where our tissues break down and returns to the ether or as Shakespeare wrote in Hamlet:

"O, that this too solid flesh would melt,

Thaw, and resolve itself into a dew!"

However, most of us would prefer to melt away this tension while we are still alive so we can benefit from the life enhancement that a smoother flow of Ki-energy can give. To release the body energetic requires freeing up the tension. Some therapies like massage or acupuncture can help us release some of this tension and fascial restriction.

Occasionally, this may manifest in a temporary worsening of the symptoms or flaring up. These symptoms can be very uncomfortable but will calm down and a slower approach afterwards may be necessary if treatment is to be continued in a tolerable way. It may take several sessions to fully release a fixed tension pattern in a part of the body.

There are some acupuncturists who are able to set off an energetic reaction upon needling which causes the patient to feel spontaneous shaking in their limbs or other parts of the body. This type of practice can help clear out the channels, widen the size of the channel pathways, promote a free flow of Ki in the body and release tension in the body. However, practitioners who can do this are very rare. The less well-known practice of 'spontaneous qigong' can also achieve a similar effect, but may require a teacher to guide the student.

How acupuncture can release tension - even in death

In an article in the North American Journal of Oriental Medicine: 'Is there a Role for Postmortem Acupuncture', Jeffrey Dann tells of an unusual account of his experiences performing acupuncture during a cadaver dissection course in 1997.

Jeffrey had brought along a box of needles with the intention of practicing needle insertion depths. He was interesting primarily in seeing how deep he would have to needle to penetrate the brain stem or other internal organs with specific points. One of the biggest safety concerns for acupuncturists is needling to the right depth so as to not injure any internal structures. For this reason, any opportunity to practice needling depth is greatly welcome.

For three days, the members were deeply involved in dissection work - removing the skin, opening up the muscles and cutting away areas of the body. Suddenly Jeffrey became frustrated. He had not carried out his original intent of practicing acupuncture needling on any of the cadavers. He felt he was missing his opportunity. So he finally pulled out an acupuncture needle looking for anywhere to test his needle depth.

He decided to insert the needle into a cadaver they had named Lucy. Lucy had died from a heart aneurism - a heart attack. During the dissection, Jeffrey had felt that Lucy had an "air of sadness" around her. Fittingly and without warning the others, he inserted the needle into her Heart 7 Acupuncture point on the wrist crease. This is a point that relate to the heart organ, but which also influences the emotions.

A flush of energy

As he inserted the needle, Jeffrey suddenly felt a flush of energy – a kind of "embarrassment heat" come over him. But more than that, one of the other members of the group, who was working on a different part of Lucy at the same time, felt a strange sensation – "a zing" rush though him and an awareness of energy running through the centre of Lucy's body down from the chest. To make things stranger, a third member suddenly remarked "I can feel it". This member too had felt a strange energetic sensation, when the needle had gone in.

At this point, the dissectors had been rocked out of convention. They all three decided to experiment with acupuncture needling on the other cadavers to see if they would experience any other unusual sensations. And indeed they did.

On the second cadaver, who they named Eve, one of the dissectors placed her hands on Eve's body and closed her eyes. Jeffrey inserted a needle between the Kidney 3 and Liver 3 Acupuncture points in the foot. Once again, the members felt a "clear and marked feeling of energy moving" and feelings of heat.

On the third cadaver, named Red, they took their experiments further. One of the dissectors held one of Red's kidneys across the room. Jeffrey then needled the sole of Red's foot on his Kidney 1 Acupuncture point. On this particular cadaver, Red had died of kidney disease so this related acupuncture point would have been significant. Here is the account:

> "John places his gloved hands on Red's Kidneys. Jeffrey places a needle at Kidney 1 on the sole of Red's foot...John says he feels "it" across the room. Doubt and excitement mix in a heady broth.

> The implications of this stagger us all. Leland suggests we were releasing stored energy in the bones and fascia. "I don't know" I say. I know this sounds really weird, but it seems as if she, wherever that is, actually carried a charge and its removal (*by acupuncture needling*) has freed her."

All of these dissectors were educated professionals. A few were either Rolfers (a type of body work therapist) or an acupuncturist like Jeffrey. Because of this, their physical senses would be well attuned.

This final remark by Leland is relevant - "That whatever that is, actually carried a charge and its removal has freed her". It reflects what I have written in this chapter about tension being held in the tissues and organs of the body and being a cause of sickness.

Various factors or emotions create tension in our body, which blocks the flow of Ki-energy, enervating our physical energies, making us weaker and contributing to sickness. Acupuncture needling has the potential to release this tension or in other words - to free us.

This experience did prompt Jeffrey to ask the questions - does acupuncture have a role in the rituals and practice of death? And is there a place for post-mortem acupuncture for people who have died in trauma or in great emotional distress as though to release the spirit.

*****

Even in stages of terminal illness or life limiting conditions, when I worked in hospice care, I saw how needling was able to help some of these patients enter a state of deep relaxation and deal with their condition better.

One of my colleagues also achieved some powerful emotional breakthroughs with patients suffering high levels of anger and resentment for their illness. Over a course of massage and acupuncture treatments, some patients are able to find a greater peace and acceptance within themselves and with the world. This prompts the idea that it is better to release and free ourselves as early as we can.

Shaking up the body holding pattern

Acupuncture needling into the body disturbs the body's holding pattern. It is as if tension is suddenly released. Signs of release are the breathing becoming deeper and the patient becoming more relaxed and contemplative. Sometimes the patient falling asleep is a good sign. In this way, tension is released and the body is given a prod into recreating a better pattern of letting go of tension.

A more notable effect of when stored tension has been released, is that the patient may feel an improvement in their mood – they feel good. Energy levels may also increase – this is partly because holding tension in the body uses up energy. Suddenly there is new energy for healing.

Be aware that after building up the energy it may also be necessary to use the energy to remove more deeper entrenched tension in the body which can result in a temporary worsening of the symptoms and tiredness again. This kind of tiredness should be differentiated from the kind of tiredness when over-treatment occurs.

A loose supple body like that of a long-term yoga practitioner or dancer is closer to an ideal state of health. But tension is not just the physical. It is also the mental and emotional. Mental tension leads to physical tension. Physical tension leads to mental tension.

Anger, resentment, jealousy are all immaterial thoughts, but can affect the physical. Anger can lead to digestive problems such as Irritable Bowel Syndrome (IBS) or migraine. Resentment leads to a lower immune system. All can lead to disturbed sleep, fatigue and a corresponding lowering of our mood.

If certain physical problems or mental emotional feelings are felt over a long period of time, there is a more noticeable effect. The long-term depressed person will have sunken chest and slumped shoulders. The angry person will have high blood pressure and palpitations. I have encountered many patients who have told me that the onset or worsening of a serious illness, whether it is a new cancer diagnosis or the onset of MS, occurred very shortly after a traumatic situation such as the bereavement of a close family member or immediately following a physical assault. Such events may act as triggers.

The word 'tension' and the word 'stress' are almost synonymous. Stress causes tension in the body. Tension stresses the body and mind. In life, it is almost impossible to eradicate tension and stress. To do so, would be akin to becoming the boy in the bubble. Safe and protected from pathogens, germs and noxious substances and yet completely cut off from life and people.

Life would be safe and sanitized but unfortunately it would be extremely boring. You are not really participating in it. This leads to frustration and then anger and consequently more tension.

Enjoyment of life is dependent on dealing with stresses in our life and eradicating their effects on our organism. It is not about removing stresses from our lives. Such a thing is unnatural, but it is about developing resilience and our ability to *weather* stresses when they come.

CHAPTER ELEVEN

THE ONSEN EXPERIENCE

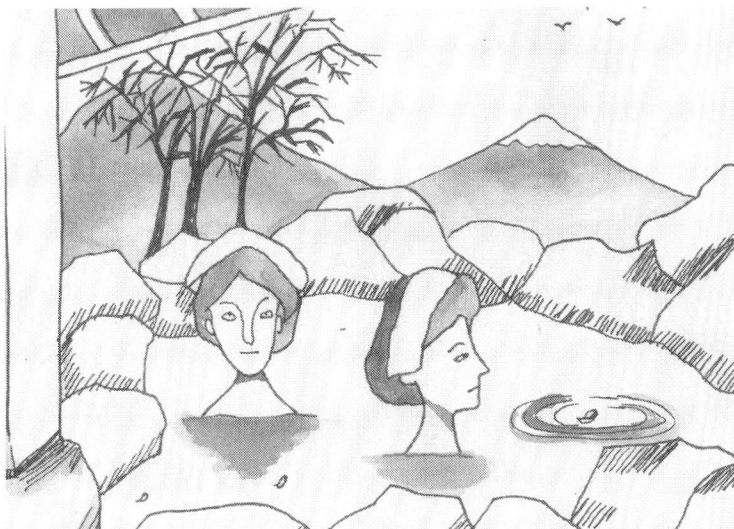

Traditional Japanese onsen - hot spring water baths in areas of natural beauty. A great way to release tension.

What is Onsen?

If you ever ask a Japanese person – what do you like to do on holiday? A common answer is - going to an onsen. Visiting onsen is a popular pastime.

Onsen are hot springs baths. As Japan sits on several active and inactive volcanoes and tectonic plate fault lines, there are plenty of hot spring areas, most of which have been cultivated into public baths.

Throughout Japan, many ryokan (travel inns) provide onsen. There are also large public baths in towns and cities. The temperature of the water in onsen is usually maintained in the range between 37 – 40°C so they are quite hot and it is this heat that really provides some benefits for the body.

Onsen is a unique experience in that you must first cleanse the body before entering, and then you enter completely naked. You are allowed a little towel for modesty. Male and female baths are separated for decency and respectful behavior towards others is expected at all times.

This helps create social cohesion and can bind a society together. By entering an area completely naked in the company of complete strangers requires trust and respect for others, which gives us another example of how the Japanese have such a strong respect for society and a strong personal identity.

Benefits of Onsen

Onsen has several benefits. Apart from physically cleansing the body, the higher temperature increases the circulation of blood and lymph and relaxes the muscles. This speeds up metabolism and detoxes the body. The act of immersing yourself in warm comfortable water is like being reborn and creates a state of relaxation and having an empty mind. You are in the moment.

Different onsens in areas of Japan also specialise in having baths that are good for specific conditions. For example, some onsen baths have water containing minerals that are good for conditions like arthritis. Others have baths that are good for purifying the skin.

Toru Abo, a Japanese research scientist who specialised in studying the immune system even goes as far to advise the use of onsen as a therapy in cases of cancer because he believes the elevated temperature of the water helps enhance the immune system.

Hot Bath Cure

In Toru Abo's book – Your Immune Revolution and Healing your Healing Power, a chapter by Kazuko Tatsumura Hillyer, PhD states:

"A Japanese theory that has existed for thousands of years states that in order to be healthy, our inner body heat must be kept high. We believe that when the inner body temperature is low, cells are deprived of heat, which is energy, and that this prevents the cells and organs from functioning well. Based on this theory, the Japanese have developed many methods for raising heat and body temperature in order to heat the body's deeper areas.

It's interesting to learn that Dr Abo recently explained this through his scientific discovery that "a person with low body temperature can't activate the lymphocytes in his white blood cells; therefore, his immune system can't function well, even if he has enough lymphocytes and white blood cells." This is why people with a low body temperature get sick easily."

In this book, factors that cause low body temperature are identified as being a lack of exercise, poor diet and eating habits, stress, drugs, smoking and excess coffee consumption, drinking too much water and an irregular lifestyle.

Two methods of increasing the internal body temperature are moxibustion therapy, which I discussed earlier, and using an onsen. Tatsumura writes:

"In Japan, we have traditional *onsen* (hot mineral spring) cures, in which we go to hot spring areas and take multiple hot mineral spring baths for a number of days… This is one of the very best ways to balance the autonomic nervous system.

When you warm your body, you stimulate the elimination of body waste through the skin, stool, and urine; stimulate digestion; relax the muscles; and relieve physiological stress."

Tatsumura does warn that hot baths (41.6°C / 107°F) are not suitable for people with high blood pressure or heart conditions. Although it can be beneficial for people with arthritis.

Onsen removes tension

Onsen is a unique Japanese experience which reinvigorates, refreshes and relaxes the body.

In my previous chapters, I discussed how stress hinders our Ki flow and causes tension in the body, which restricts the flow of Ki energy. One useful method of relaxing this tension and stress is with heat. The heat from immersing yourself in a hot onsen bath can help to relax the muscles, enhance the blood and lymph circulation, and improve the flow of Ki in the body.

Immersing yourself in the hot water of onsen literally melts away tension and hardness from the muscles.

Unfortunately, in the West, hot spring baths are not so common. So, the next best thing is to take hot baths at home. Epsom salts can also be added to the water to enhance the effects

If you are walking around with a hard shell of a body carrying all of your life, family and work stresses in your musculature, it would be beneficial to take regular hot baths as an adjunct to your health program. If you visit Japan, you must also try the onsen experience.

CHAPTER TWELVE

BENEFITS OF MEDITATION

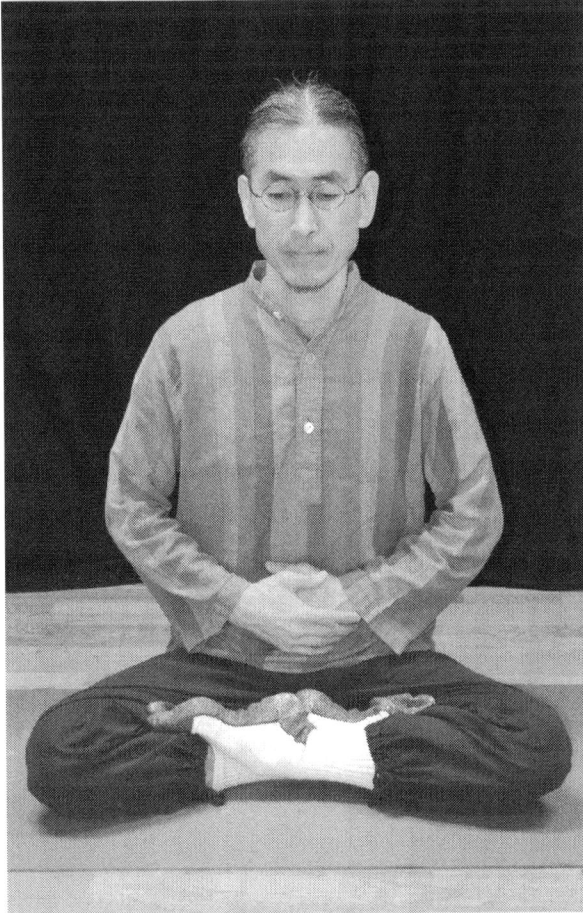

Meditation: The Meditative Zone

Meditation, the practice of stilling the mind and body and turning inwards is one of the simplest yet most powerful ways to improve emotional wellbeing. The West is externally focused. It is more yang in nature, which tends to view the solution to any problem as coming from outside the body such as a pharmaceutical drug, surgery or consultation with a health expert.

Daily meditation can be simply described as 'sitting doing nothing'. By switching off external stimuli and focusing the mind inwards, meditation activates a state of recharge and mental cleansing.

At first it is difficult and the mind wanders madly from one thought to another, but meditation acts like the shining of a spotlight on your mind. You see how the mind operates, its constant activity and how it moves turbulently like the waves of a ship in a storm flowing from one thought to another, engaging in one emotional state over another. Over time, it will calm.

Whereas activity and movement is yang, meditation and sleep, which are both restorative activities are yin. Even activities where we do not physically move the body, but instead use and strain the mental faculties such as doing computer work or studying can be considered yang activities.

I have felt more drained spending 8 hours doing administrative work, phone calls, emails and spreadsheets then doing work that involves physical movement such as lifting and moving. It is important to balance external yang activities with yin meditation

There are many different ways to meditate, from focusing the mind on one thing such as the breath, or a single point like a flame, an icon like Jesus or Buddha or focusing it on one of the body's chakras. I prefer to simply sit without doing anything, not trying to achieve or un-achieve anything, just simply sit and be quiet, sometimes watching the thoughts without trying to change them.

Ultimately, after some time, it is possible to fall into a 'meditative zone', a state of relaxation where your interest in the external environment decreases and you melt into a calm relaxed internal state. It is possible that in this state, the sensation of energy flow in the body may be perceived.

The meditative zone helps calm the body down and make a person less easily riled up when faced with daily annoying occurrences like stress at work, relationship strife or bureaucratic nuisances. It is a useful tool if you live in a busy city with lots of pressures.

A State of Relaxation

Although you may be exerting some muscle tension to hold a meditative pose such as keeping the back muscles and spine straight, overall the body is in a peak state of relaxation.

It is different to the kind of relaxation that is experienced when flopping on a deckchair on the beach or in a Jacuzzi. It is a conscious state of relaxation which also allows you to scan your body with your mind to seek out tense areas or patterns of tension in areas like the shoulders, abdomen, hands, neck or any part of the body and then to consciously let go of that tension to rewrite this holding pattern, Meditation helps to re-educate the body.

Sitting meditation

In either seiza or cross-legged position, hold the spine straight, tuck the chin slightly in and keep the tongue at the roof of the mouth. Close the eyes or keep them half open and hold the pose for 5-10 minutes. Perform this exercise once or twice a day.

Standing meditation

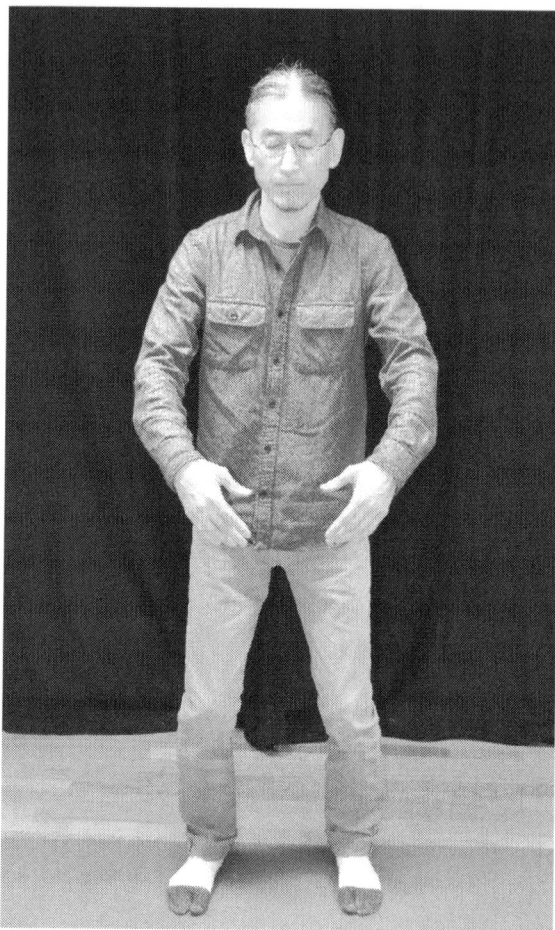

This Chinese qigong exercise can be considered a form of standing meditation. This pose has the benefit of opening up all of the channel pathways in the body to encourage a smooth flow of Ki-energy.

- Stand with legs shoulder width apart.

- Slightly bend the knees.

- Either keep arms by your side or imagine that you holding a ball in front of you.

- Keep the spine straight, tuck the chin slightly in.

- Close or keep the eyes half open and simply stand for 5 to 15 minutes or more.

- Carry out this exercise 1 or 2 times a day.

Lying meditation

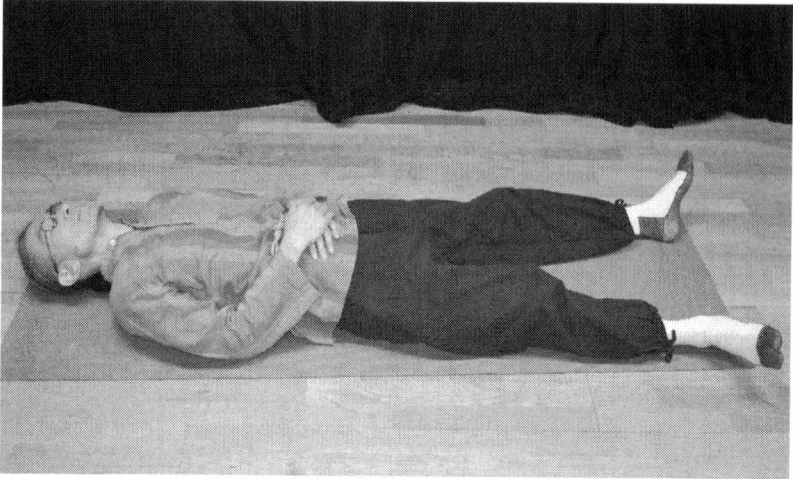

If you are feeling unwell, tired or are recovering from an illness, this is a good pose. Simply lie straight. Uncross the legs and keep them a little apart. Place your hands on either side and open with palms upwards or place them on your hara (abdomen). Consciously relax and release any tension in your body.

A flat firm surface like a yoga mat on a wooden floor or carpet is good because it will help to lengthen your spine however, a bed or sofa is acceptable. Focus on breathing into your lower abdomen in relaxed deep breaths. This pose can be held for longer periods of 10-30 minutes.

Daily life meditation poses

After you have practiced the above poses for some time, you may start to become acquainted with the subtle energetic flows that can occur in the body. You may find it possible to slip into the same 'meditative zone' whilst relaxing during normal times of the day such as sitting and reading a newspaper or even during walking.

The meditative zone & healing

The 1970s TV drama, Kung Fu, stars David Carradine as a Kung Fu monk travelling through the Wild West of America. Along the way, he faces various challenges. In one episode, he is captured by a gang of bandits and imprisoned with another young cowboy. They are both held captive in significant discomfort.

The cowboy notices that David is unusually calm and asks what he is doing. David tells him that he is meditating. The cowboy asks for him to teach him the method which he so does, and the cowboy is able to get through the night. After they part, the cowboy endeavors to continue his practice of meditation.

Though it is a TV series, there are some who believe that sicknesses can be healed with the power of meditation. A colleague of mine who travelled to China to study under some Masters, found that meditation made up a large part of their practice. When he asked for their advice on how to recover from a long-term, health problem he was suffering from, he was simply told: "You must meditate more".

I mentioned earlier about the 'meditative zone'. In this zone, it is possible to become aware of waves of energy, ripples or vibrations moving throughout your body. It is a place, where if I am suffering some physical discomfort, some of these sensations can be reduced. I believe this zone is potentially healing if it is practiced for prolonged periods of time, though I make no promises.

The simple thing about the zone, is that it requires no particular work to enter. Just a quiet space where you simply sit doing nothing. It is also better to enter it by sitting in seiza or cross-legged position. In the beginning, it may take many repeated sessions of meditation practice until you become aware of the zone.

CHAPTER THIRTEEN

EMOTIONS

心

Kokoro

Heart & Mind

Humans are highly emotional creatures. Though we may fill our days with practical work and obligations with things like preparing or acquiring food, earning money, looking after the physical needs of others – children parents, sick family members, commuting, studying or other general activities, there is an emotional undercurrent running through many of our actions.

If we are having a difficult situation, that undercurrent may be anger or anxiety. If we have excessive financial stresses - that undercurrent may be anxiety or worry. The loss of a loved one - leaves us feeling deeply sad inside. Being over-pressured or facing some kind of workplace stress brings irritation – another form of anger. So-called 'failures' in life - a failed exam, job loss or ridicule from others may bring depression. Gaining a huge amount of money from investing in the stock market may bring over-excitement.

For the most part, we try not to allow other people to see these emotions. We keep them hidden – we wear masks. Western societies do not encourage people to be truthful about their feelings. The standard question "how are you?" is never meant to be answered honestly.

One of the reasons is that a lot of people are holding all sorts of hurts inside. We are meant to put these aside and get on with life. It is only when people face a tragic loss, or are facing a terminal illness that they are allowed to talk about the feelings and emotions to 'sanctioned' listeners called counselors. Although in some cases, this is too late.

Experiencing our emotions is part of the human experience. Emotions have a powerful energy, which can never be destroyed. Their energy can only be transmuted. To shut them off, to try to suppress them only causes them to bubble and boil within us until eventually they attack our own tissues or explode periodically in disruptive outbursts, violence or distort our personality and make us become *weird*.

Emotions are our antennas. They bring forth colour and feeling to all our life experiences. Some emotions are perceived as 'negative' like anger, depression, and sadness. Some are seen as 'positive' like joy. But actually, there is no negative or positive. We either express them healthily or we overuse or misuse them and express them harmfully onto ourselves or other people. In this section, we will look at emotions and ways of expressing them healthily.

*****

病は気から

Yamai wa Ki kara

Sickness comes from the mind and feelings

This Japanese proverb – 'sickness comes from the mind and feelings', considers that health and sickness can be caused by our emotional state.

Traditional Chinese Medicine and the Emotions

The Ancient Chinese recognized that emotions can be a cause of illness. In particular, the emotions of sadness, anger, worry, fear and joy.

Sadness

Stagnation of Ki-energy flow in the body can be caused by emotional distress. Sadness or grief *pulls* the Ki-energy inwards. We see this in depressed people with shoulders hunched forward and head hanging downwards, which hinders the flow of Ki-energy in the chest area.

As an experiment, if you take on this pose, you'll notice that it affects your mental state as well and physically restricts the volume of breath you can take.

Over a long time, this depression of the Ki-energy will show itself in the voice. The voice may take on a subtle tone of sadness or a crying-like quality to it. In acupuncture, emphasis is put on listening diagnosis of the speech and tone to pick up on the qualities of the voice.

Sadness relates to the Lung Channel. The connection is more apparent, if we consider that a depressed or sad person with a slumped chest has a posture which naturally restricts the lung organ and the flow of Ki-energy in the Lung channel.

The antidote is to stretch our chests and do deep breathing or regular exercise to get the lungs working. It is well known that regular exercise can help with depression.

Anger

Anger makes the energy fly upwards and outwards. If we observe people caught up in the heat of arguing, we see flushed red faces and lots of arm flailing as well as puffing up of chests and shouting. The energy is moving upwards and outwards. We need only see TV shows like the Jeremy Kyle show or EastEnders to see how ugly it makes us appear as humans.

Worse, is that anger is like a raging fire burning out of control in a small town made of wooden houses. It grows, consuming and destroying everything in its path. Anger is strangely addictive and two angry people arguing together will feed each other's anger with their fire. In some ways, it is like a kind of madness and can lead to violence such as the 'crime of passion' or 'provocation' in legal cases. Fortunately, one person usually backs down in arguments, but that anger still remains within causing harm.

In Traditional Chinese Medicine, Anger relates to the Liver channel, which is classified as Wood in the 5-phase theory of the elements. Wood burns and fuels fire. When anger starts to flare, it is best to take a time out, take some deep breaths and escape the situation before you really lose your temper and anger takes a hold. This is especially the case for men where anger can lead to physical violence, although it can be equally applicable to women.

Alcohol and anger are terrible combinations and will lead to self-destruction. Regular meditative type exercises and a wholesome diet with lots of green foods and wholegrains and limiting the amount of meat you eat can help pacify the liver and help modify our anger response.

In the book - 'The Only Two Causes of All Diseases' Toru Abo talks about the harmful effects of anger on the body and how it puts the body in a state of low oxygen level (hypoxia) and coldness (hypothermia), which he believes are risk factors in the development of cancer.

For example, he says:

> "Imagine when you have bursts of anger. You are naturally holding your breath when you get angry. When we continue to hold our breath the amount of blood flow into the veins will be limited. This will lead to hypothermia".

Toru also notes that anger can recede if we let it. He gives the example of a boss losing his temper at an employee:

> "Remember that bursts of anger last for about three minutes at the longest. You don't need to be twisted around your boss's finger or further fuel new bursts of anger by talking back. Leave an angry person alone for 30 minutes and they will lose the energy to stay angry".

This is good advice for anyone in a relationship. Husband and wife arguments can be particularly pernicious because they live together and their boundaries are more intertwined. Arguments and minor irritations are a normal course of affairs.

However, for a more harmonious life, if one person is feeling irritable, it is best to avoid getting sucked into an argument. It is far safer to withdraw, go for a walk to the shop, walk the dog, clean the car - anything. Try to allow the other person some space to calm down, then a potentially heated and stressful situation can be averted.

Arguments are like fires. They burn and burn out of control consuming anything combustible around them. If there is no fuel such as another person to feed the argument, they can die down.

Sometimes, anger and irritability is chronic and not easily avoided such as a bullying workplace or abusive relationship. Toru warns:

> "Living in a lifestyle where you snap at people easily is harmful for your interpersonal relationships. It is also harmful to the cells in your own body".

Worry

Worry knots the qi. When something bothers us such as an un-payable bill, work problem, health problem or difficult family relationship, we worry about it. The issue goes around and around in our head as we imagine the worst. It can send us in a loop as we keep thinking the same thoughts and imagining the worst.

It is a kind of mental sickness. This type of thinking pattern *knots* the Ki-energy flow in our body. Our body clocks go off; we find it hard to settle at night and can't sleep. We start waking up at night and sleeping in late. Our energy declines and we start craving sugary foods or we simply lose our appetites. Excessive worry causes a slow weakening of our body's Ki making us more susceptible to illness.

Fear

Fear can come in many forms. We will all experience some kind of fear in our lives. For example, fear of exam failure, fear of job loss, fear of rejection by someone you like, fear of a presentation, speech or job interview. These are natural challenges we go through, which are part of human experience.

But it is the more extreme forms of fear that are very harmful for our health. Growing up in a war zone produces extreme fear. We fear for our safety and the safety of our family members. So too can being exposed to prolific bullying at school or living with an abusive husband, which creates daily fear. Fear harms the Kidney Channel and kidney organ in Traditional Chinese medicine. It makes the Ki-energy flow downwards.

One simple way to understand this is when someone is suddenly shocked or terrified and they wet themselves or have diarrhoea (Ki flowing downwards). I have treated people who have experienced domestic abuse. It is apparent to me that the stresses they went though were significant factors in their presenting health problem. To overcome a fearful situation requires courage and perseverance as well as support from others.

Joy

Joy may seem an unusual cause of disease but if we think of joy as 'over stimulation', then it makes sense. For example, Traditional Chinese medicine says that excess joy damages the heart.

If we consider the Type A personality - impatient, competitive and uptight - a type of person who may work on a busy trading floor, shouting into a cell phone, drugged up with blood pressure pills and cocaine, we know that this type is severely over-stimulated and is also at greater risk of a heart attack.

'Joy' and overstimulation comes in many forms. The gambler addicted to the races, casino or online poker is afflicted by Joy. Joy also affects the young clubber taking ecstasy or amphetamine and partying all night. Even the sex-addicted celebrity who is able to indulge all their desires without limit will be afflicted by an over-stimulation of the senses (Joy).

In some ways, Joy is the most harmful of the emotions because of its addictive nature. Unsurprisingly, in Traditional Chinese medicine, Joy damages the Heart Channel and organ.

The antidote to Joy is to regulate the heart. Celebrities are a good example of the dangers of excess joy because with their disproportionate wealth, they are able to live like kings and are in fact encouraged to indulge in all the temptations that money and fame can buy

Compare the hedonistic lifestyles of people like the British footballer George Best or the musician Prince, with the more balanced life of the actor and practicing Buddhist, Richard Gere. Regular meditation practice as well as developing a sense of appreciation and gratitude for what we do have in life can counteract the addictive quality of joy.

Moderating our desires also helps. Desire is one of the driving forces behind our need for joy. In the history of our species, desire has always been a potential pitfall, ever since Eve was tempted by the Snake to eat of the tree of knowledge of good and evil. Since the 1960s, desire has been ramped up as a driving force. The desire for self-indulgence, materialism, money, sex and pleasure has been toxic for our society leaving a large financial and spiritual debt which must be paid for by future generations.

Desire underpins the drive for joy. Desire is recognized as a cause of disease in traditional Chinese Taoist folklore as seen in this quote from the book 'Seven Taoist Masters. A Folk Novel of China'.

> "If you want to get rid of the sickness of spirit and body, you must get to its cause. If you know the cause, then you will know the cure. The primary cause of ill health is none other than craving.
>
> Craving creates the obstacles to health. These obstacles are desire for liquor, sexual desire, greed for riches, and bad temper. Those who wish to cultivate health and longevity must first remove these obstacles."

But how do you go about reducing craving and desire. The book answers:

> "To eradicate the four obstacles to health-liquor, sexual desire, riches, and bad temper-one must cultivate the heart. Once the heart is tamed, the cause of ill health will disappear".

This book also talks about meditation, which as we discussed is a useful tool that can help to tame the heart, reduce desire and regulate Joy.

Stress in Oriental Medicine: The emotions

We discussed earlier about stress and tension in the body. Stress or tension can also be caused by the emotions. Usually, stress causes a stagnation of Ki-energy flow. It over-stimulates the Liver organ and creates a corresponding imbalance in the flow of Ki-energy in the Liver Channel leading to Liver Ki stagnation.

Stressful experiences cause an over-expression of certain emotions in the human body which can impact the body negatively.

The emotions related to stress are typically anger and irritation, which affects the Liver Channel. Worry, which affects the Spleen Channel. Depression - affecting the Liver and Spleen. Fear, which affects the Kidney and Sadness, which affects the Lung.

In this way stress has the potential to affect the entire body system in Chinese medicine and it is up to the trained acupuncturist to decide which system is most affected and which emotion is most prominent and treat accordingly. However, by far the most active organ in stress is the Liver.

Analogies

The ancient Chinese liked to use analogies to describe how the body works and one way was to define the organs as members of the government.

The Heart being the most important was called the Emperor. The Liver is traditionally called the General of the organ system. And if you imagine the General of the armed forces, we envision a strong official – one that keeps the Empire (the body) safe and stable.

However, when the General is under pressure (perhaps by an attacking army) the General may well become short tempered and lash out at its subordinates.

It may well order the farmers (think - digestive system) to stop growing food and take up arms so that no new food is grown.

It may well bully all the ministers and advisors (other organs) to stop their duties and bend their will to his own.

At worse he may well plan a coup against the Emperor and take over the empire with a brutal dictatorship. This is an analogy, but metaphorically this is what happens in the human body.

The Liver becomes over-active. It is one of the most powerful organs in the body and it has the power to affect everything else. When stressed, it may well overexert itself on the digestive system (the spleen and stomach) causing digestive problems, diarrhoea, constipation gas or IBS. It may well overact on the lungs causing a worsening of conditions like asthma.

The Liver controls the gynecological system in women along with the Kidneys and can cause painful or irregular periods. It can even stop fertility. It can affect the heart (which governs sleep) causing bad dreams and insomnia. The Liver also sends energy upwards in the body causing headaches or migraine.

One reason that stressed people drink alcohol is that it has a depressive effect on the liver and helps calm it down although at the same time stimulating it in the long term. In this respect, although alcohol can help in the short term, it can make things worse and lead to addiction in the long term.

Fortunately, there are things you can do to calm the overactive Liver down by yourself and help to reclaim balance in your life allowing you to deal with the stress in your life with a level head.

Interventions such as acupuncture or massage can help to rebalance the overactive Liver energy and regulate the stress response. However, another way to calm or quieten the General (Liver) is to strengthen the Emperor (Heart).

Give the Emperor more power and the General has to obey. Meditation strengthens the Heart. In this way meditation can be a potent way particularly if you meditate on the Heart chakra energy field (right between the breast area).

The colour green is also associated with the Liver and can help calm it down. This can be in the form of eating green leafy vegetables – cabbage, spinach, kale or going for regular walks in the park. Even having plants in the house can have a calming effect on the body.

青葉は目の薬

Aoba wa me no kusuri

Greenery is Medicine for the Eyes

This Japanese proverb – 'greenery is medicine for the eyes', reflects the importance of nature on our health.

The Japanese refer to trees, forests and plants as greenery. As Japan is a mountainous country, a common pastime is to go mountain walking, followed sometimes by a trip to the onsen (hot spring bath). There are many mountains of various sizes in Japan. Some can easily be climbed in a few hours or there is the active volcano Mount Fuji.

Whilst living in Tokyo, I climbed up Mountain Takao several times and was always struck by the number of elderly Japanese men and women I would pass along the way, who clearly were very healthy. Along the way, there are many trees and plants - plenty of medicine for the eyes. Walking up the mountain was a very calming experience for me, so much so that I would go hiking up there as often as I could.

In Traditional Chinese Medicine, the Liver is related to the eyes in the human body. Our modern world overuses the eyes through looking at TV, the internet, smart phones and computer work. All this over-stimulates the eyes and overworks the Liver. Again, the antidote to this is by closing our eyes through meditation and tuning our senses inwards. These are just small steps you can take, but even small changes can lead to significant improvements in the long term.

CHAPTER FOURTEEN

FOOD AND DIET

The topic of food and health has probably become one of the most complex and contradictory areas concerning health. There are many different ideas, viewpoints, diet plans as well as various corporate and industrial forces which have turned what should be a simple thing into a complicated topic.

For example, if you see a Western scientific 'dietician', a healthy diet is based on consuming adequate amounts of the recommended daily allowance (RDA) of carbohydrates, proteins, fibre, vitamins and minerals.

It does not necessarily matter whether the carbohydrates and vitamins comes from fortified sugary cereal or from sweet potatoes. With a certain degree of opposition, there are the various schools of 'nutritionist', which are generally more imaginative with diets and may promote a more *natural* diet based on the consumption of vegetables, pulses, whole-grains and lean meats along with various supplements.

Then there are the more specialist nutritionists or naturopaths that may promote certain ways of eating with an emphasis on certain food groups such as high fibre diets, low carbohydrate diets, anti-candida diets, fasting, food combining or raw food diets. And of course, there are the weight loss diets. Diets designed to make us lose weight.

There are so many diets. Just to name a few – there is the palaeolithic diet, the food combining diet, the weightwatchers diet, the F plan, the exclusion diet, the zone diet, the Atkins diet, the Okinawa diet, the Eskimo diet, the Dukan diet, the apple a day diet, the banana diet, the grapefruit diet, the South beach diet, the cabbage soup diet, juice fasting, the specific carbohydrate diet, the gluten free diet, the warrior diet, the alkaline diet, the blood type diet, the Dr Hay diet, the macrobiotic diet, the candida diet, the high protein diet, the low protein diet, the high carbohydrate diet, the low carbohydrate diet, the French women don't get fat diet, the low glycemic index diet, raw foodism, the sugar busters diet, there's even a junk food diet.

The list is endless. Most of them are related to losing weight but some of them are about improving a health condition or simply to improve general health. Maybe, just as the final curtain is drawn on the last of human civilisation, there will have been as many diet plans in existence as there are stars in the sky.

As expected, Traditional Oriental Medicine also has its own take on food. In the Traditional Chinese Medicine (TCM) system of Oriental medicine, food is classified with different energetic qualities.

They can be heating – they put heat in the body. Or cooling – in that they cool the body. They may also be damp forming - causing phlegm, mucous or weight gain. Some foods increase the yang energy of the body and others nourish the yin. Some foods may be considered neutral. Basically, all food has energetic qualities, which affect the body in different ways.

Foods that are considered heating are spices, red meat and lamb. Cooling foods are typically raw foods like cucumber, eggplant and raw fish. Damp forming foods are dairy, oil and sugar.

Some foods strengthen or weaken certain organs. For example, the sweet taste affects the spleen and stomach, which governs the digestive system. Naturally sweet foods like grains – both white and brown strengthens the spleen and stomach. However, excessively sweet foods like refined sugar, candies and cakes can weaken it.

The yin and yang of foods has many aspects and is not altogether that simple. One way of looking at yin foods is that they increase the yin aspects of the body like the blood and flesh. Therefore, proteins like meat and fish may be considered yin. Foods that increase energy quickly may be considered yang such as alcohol or refined sugar. However, as discussed in the article on yin and yang, everything is relative. So, for example, although meat may generally be considered yin due to the density of protein they contain, red meats are considered more yang than white meats like chicken.

Foods are grouped by colour according to the theory of Five elements. For example, the colour white is said to resonate with the metal element and in particular the lung and large intestine – so white colour foods like cauliflower or white rice may be beneficial to the lungs. Green strengthens the wood element – the liver, so green leafy vegetables may be beneficial to the liver.

Foods are grouped by shape. The kidney bean resembles the human kidney and so is said to strengthens the kidneys. Walnuts look like the brains and are said to strengthens the brain.

Like fixes like. Offal meat like animal liver, kidney and intestines are said to nourish the corresponding human equivalent organ. Pig blood (Black pudding) can nourish human blood.

Foods are classified by action. For example, spicy foods encourage perspiration and sweating. If we have stagnant energy such as having poor circulation or being overweight – then some spicy foods can move the circulation and encourage the opening of the pores. However, this can be a quick fix to the underlying problem as too much yang (spicy foods) can eventually lead to too much yin (mucous, phlegm and excess weight) in the body, undermining it.

Damp forming foods cause damp in the body. Damp can be thought of as phlegm or mucus. Some people are intolerant to dairy or wheat and when they eat it they may find a buildup of phlegm and mucus in the throat or even in the stool.

How foods are cooked also affects their energetic qualities. For example, fried, barbecued and grilled cooking methods, use intense heat for a shorter period of cooking time and has a searing effect on the food. These methods are considered to be more yang compared to boiling or steaming, which tends to soften the food and is considered a more yin method. In particular, frying or deep-fat frying has both a yang-heating and damp-forming effect on food due to the combination of heat and oil (a damp food).

Deep fat fried foods may be very hard for people with weak digestive systems to digest. An excess of this kind of food can lead to what in TCM is described as damp heat in the body. Damp heat refers to any kind of puss-filled inflammation or painful inflammation.

We see this in the adolescent fast food employee who eats free hamburgers and fries every day for lunch and suffers from cystic acne. We see this in the middle-aged person who eats fried rump steaks, ribs and fried chicken frequently and suffers from swollen joints.

A historical example of damp heat would be the condition of gout – a painful arthritic condition, which affects the foot. It was called the "king of diseases and the disease of kings" or "the rich man's disease". King Henry VIII was known to suffer from this 'damp-heat' condition no doubt caused by his excess diet of rich foods and alcohol.

There are other principles – a little of one flavour can strengthen an organ or body function. So a little sweet (from grains) can strengthen the spleen and stomach. A little of the bitter flavour - strengthens the heart; a little pungent strengthens the lung, sour strengthens the liver, salty strengthens the kidneys.

However, too much of a flavour can weaken the same organ. Too much sugar (refined sugar) weakens the Spleen and Stomach (organs associated with digestion). Too much of the pungent flavour (curry) weakens the lungs. Some people after eating strong curry may get a lot of mucus in their throat afterwards.

There is a debate over raw and cooked foods. In Chinese food therapy, it is recommended to cook foods. This contrasts with the Western raw food movement - especially popular in California, which claims that the cooking process 'denatures' food and destroys raw enzymes. However, not everyone can tolerate raw foods.

Raw foods can lead to stomach aches and excess flatulence in people with less than robust digestive systems. It may work in a hot dry state like California, but not so well in a cold damp country like England.

Other issues are vegetarianism and fasting. Despite the proximity of India and China and the transfer of ideas which had gone on for centuries between the two countries, there are some fundamental differences concerning eating habits and diet. In traditional Indian medicine, fasting (the abstinence of food for a short period of time) is practiced to rest the digestive system and to detoxify the body. However, in Chinese dietetics, fasting is discouraged as it is seen as weakening the digestive system. Instead simple, plain, easy digestible foods and herbal teas are recommended for sickness.

Vegetarianism is also a common part of the Indian diet. However, with the exception of Taoists and monks, the Chinese are not generally vegetarian. Meat strengthens both the yang and yin and is seen as an essential part of a healthy diet. In the Chinese diet, mealtimes are generally a combination of vegetables, meats, fish, rice or noodles.

This doesn't mean that the Indians are right and the Chinese wrong or the other way around. Both means of eating convey benefits and disadvantages to these people. What this teaches us is that there are no hard and fast rules when it comes to food and eating habits.

A more important factor is that good digestion depends not just on the quality of the food we eat, but also on our ability to digest it. If our digestion is impaired, we will not absorb the useful nutrients from it.

In Chinese medicine, the Spleen and Stomach meridians and organs control digestion. If they are weak, then we may suffer from low energy and other symptoms such as feeling bloated or tiredness after eating, rumbling in the intestines, diarrhea and aches in the stomach or food intolerances. Food may not be properly absorbed causing low energy and a thin body.

Conversely, food may be too well absorbed but not properly converted into energy in the body resulting in weight gain and again tiredness. In this way, we could eat the best food in the world and it will go to waste. When a person has strong digestion, they can eat a big mac and fries and take in benefit from it. When a person has weak digestion, they can eat a Jamie Oliver meal and gain very little benefit from it. There is a common joke – 'only sick people can be found in health food shops'.

CHAPTER FIFTEEN

THE WAY WE EAT

The way we eat, the time and the environment we eat in all affects our digestion, particularly if we feel stressed when we eat or if we eat in a rush. Some people at work will stuff a cold sandwich down their throat during a rushed five-minute break and a coca cola during the winter. This makes the body energetically cold as they are eating cold energy foods in a cold season.

The traditional Chinese have an energy circulation clock, which shows the circulation of Ki-energy through the Channels. In this clock, the morning time period of 7am to 9am is the time of maximum Stomach-Ki flow and the period of 9am to 11am is the time of maximum Spleen-Ki flow. Both these organs deal with digestion and absorption in Traditional Chinese medicine.

These four hours are considered to be the time when the digestive system is at its maximum peak of power in the Chinese clock and where it would be good to have our most substantial meal. However, it should be considered that in modern life, we do not waken with the sun nor do we do as much physical work as our ancestors.

In this way, it is probably not as necessary to eat a large breakfast during this time period. For more sedentary people, it is better to eat a light breakfast. However, a physical worker would be far better off having a large breakfast to fuel their activities for the day.

In Asian countries like Japan, traditionally they follow this way of eating by having a substantial meal for breakfast. A traditional breakfast would be a bowl of rice, miso soup, some vegetables and grilled mackerel.

In the West, breakfasts used to be more substantial. My father's generation were brought up with a large bowl of porridge oats, bread and butter and sometimes kippers. However, now there is a trend towards having lighter and quicker breakfasts.

Today, many people have a few spoonfuls of cornflakes, a slice of toast or they forego breakfast and have two to three cups of coffee and a cigarette. It may well be that the post afternoon slump and craving for snacks that many people suffer from may be attributed to an insufficient breakfast.

There is a long-term consequence to inadequate eating. Your body must use up its own resources and precious yin energy in order to provide yang energy for daily movement and activity. In short, you're selling yourself short.

Another example of Western eating habits is that the evening meal time is slowly becoming a solitary affair. Even in families with two or more members, the TV is often switched on and takes center stage. Some families eat in separate rooms.

Typically, the Chinese family sit down at the table together. Food is placed on dishes in the center and they take a small portion and place it in their bowls unlike the Western way of having their own plate filled up with everything. This way, there must be interaction between family members. Eating becomes a social event. The TV may be on in the room in the background, but it does not take central focus. Food takes central focus.

Some years ago, I was fortunate to be invited by a Chinese friend to her house for a meal with other guests for the Chinese New Year.

In typical Western fashion, I filled up my small bowl to maximum with everything I wanted. It seemed more efficient to get everything in one go, then to have to keep takings bits here and there with chopsticks. This attracted one small remark of disdain from my host. Fortunately, I was among friends. We discussed different eating habits and I was told that the Western way of filling up everything you want in a bowl or plate is seen as selfish. It was an idea I had never considered before.

I had always taken it for granted that typically we have everything we want on our own plate. When we order food in a restaurant, food comes on our own plate. We do not share it. It seems more efficient. But then by eating in this way, eating has the potential to become a selfish event.

Everything is set. We do not need to interact. We don't need to argue who's going to eat that last piece, although sometimes it can be mildly tedious if you really want to eat the last delicious piece of sushi or gyoza (Chinese dumpling) on a plate, but you don't want to look greedy, so you offer it to someone else to finish. Although, perhaps this is an exercise in selflessness.

Japan's food culture

If you switch on the TV in Japan at any time of the day, you will very likely see a programme about food or a bunch of celebrities visiting a small eatery somewhere in the country. The camera will show two or three studio members sitting down and eating the food, sometimes with a small introduction by a narrator or a small interview with the restaurant owner.

The cast will take a mouthful of the food and nearly always exclaim "Oishiiii" or "Umaiiii", which translates as 'Delicious'. The restaurant could be a small ramen noodle bar in downtown Tokyo, an expensive French restaurant in Ginza in Tokyo's uptown district or a local delicacy in Aichi prefecture. The location is not important. All that matters is that the food is of good quality, is well presented and tastes delicious.

Food is an important pastime in Japan, with numerous restaurants, bento take-out and eateries at reasonable prices everywhere. I lived in downtown Tokyo some years ago and every Sunday there was always a queue of people outside a local nondescript looking ramen shop waiting to get a seat. The place had a good reputation and yet was inexpensive due to it being in a small downtown area.

In Japan, the food choices are varied and inexpensive, with high standards of service and food quality. Even supermarkets sell take-out meals of good quality.

Part of being in Japan is experiencing the food and then wondering when you return to the UK, why it can't be the same here and at the same prices and yet, despite their love of food, the Japanese are some of the trimmest people on the planet despite having the same access to typical junk foods such as MacDonald's, KFC and a few of their own variations. There is very little obesity. The average size for a woman is 6-10 in Japan.

It may also be because the Japanese appreciate food but do not over-eat. They consume significantly less carbohydrates and fat then their Western counterparts today as an ingrained habit.

The lesson here is simple in the West. To lose weight, may not simply require *Spartan* weightwatcher-type diets or strict calorie counting. We simply need to appreciate our foods more, not overeat and eat a good balance of fish, meat, vegetables, pickles and limited amounts of carbohydrate. We also need to be more active to burn off those calories.

As an acupuncture practitioner, my advice is simple. Eat fresh and adequate amounts of vegetables, protein and carbs. Limit your intake of processed foods. Prepare and cook foods yourself. Boil, steam or grill in preference to frying.

During the cold seasons, soups and stews are nourishing. During the summer, some raw foods can be fine if your digestive system is healthy.

If you have digestive problems, cook foods softly so that they are easily digestible, and be wary of eating highly fibrous foods like cabbage, brown rice or beans. Raw foods may also be difficult to digest.

Also listen to your body – if a food or supplement upsets your gut, no matter how *healthy* it is meant to be, then maybe it's no good for you. Listen and respond to the messages your body tells you.

Be aware of the psychological nature of food. If you crave salty snacks or sweets excessively – it can be an imbalance in the body but there is also the consideration that there is a psychological reason for the craving. When we are stressed or deeply troubled, sugary and salty foods can be a way of self-medicating ourselves in much the same way that people may drink alcohol or take illicit drugs to numb themselves from the stress of life's problems.

In much the same way that factory farmed animals are effectively force-fed with whatever we choose to give them – GM grains, antibiotics, steroids or even brain material from their own species (causing Mad Cow disease due to prions), we as humans are also to various extents 'force-fed' by the food industry in collaboration with the advertising industry.

Food is a billion-dollar business and a major part of the economy. Certain industries depend for their very survival that enough of us Homo sapiens eat factory farmed chicken and pork, hamburgers, bread or milk, frosted sugar flakes or sweetened fizzy drinks on a daily basis. The last thing we are ever expected to do is to grow and eat our own food.

It is in this way, that modern humans in the developed world have lost connection with food. As food today is imported from thousands of miles away, we don't even know which foods are local to our environment. Only gardeners know which vegetables are in season.

Meat is far more easily available today than in any generation previously and we probably eat too much. We tend to forget that meat was a luxury item for our ancestors. We have forgotten that humans must still follow the natural laws if we want to thrive in health (not just survive).

A major principle is to live in tune with nature. There is a price to be paid for spending all our days in an air-conditioned room set to the same comfortable temperature in summer and winter.

In much the same way, we can buy and eat salad from the supermarket chilled section every day during the coldest period of winter. If we eat a yin food in a yin season, we make our bodies too yin. In a yin season (winter), it is better to eat a yang food (a warm stew) to balance yin and yang.

The Chinese were smart - too smart. They foresaw the damage that occurs to the body when we live out of tune with nature and found a simplistic way of expressing it. Despite our incredible advances in science, medicine and technology, we still have the same bodies as the ancients and are still subject to the same natural laws. Fortunately, their wisdom has been preserved and is waiting for us to rediscover it.

*****

腹八分に医者いらず

Hara hachibu ni isha irazu

Eat till your stomach is 8 tenths full and you will never need a doctor

This is a basic Japanese proverb, which simply means if we eat smaller portions of no more than 80% or eight-tenths of our stomach's capacity, we can remain healthy and not need to seek medical help.

In Toru Abo's book 'The Only Two causes of Disease', he discussed the origins of - 'Hara Hachi Bu Me' and the concept of eating moderately. It is also known as the 80% diet.

We often think that abundant food is a relatively modern phenomenon when we look at our supermarkets and the expanding waist lines of some people today, but the problem of overeating and essentially gluttony has been a problem for anyone who has access to plenty of food. This seems to have been the case in Japan during the Edo period.

In the 80% diet, you eat until you fill moderately full and then stop. The idea was first written by Ekiken Kaibara, a Confucian scholar of the Edo period. He lived from 1630 to 1714 and he introduced a specific diet to help maintain health called Syoku Yo Jyo. This diet was further developed by the Edo scholar Nanboku Mizuno (1757 - 1834).

The story of Nanboku goes that he was living a fast life - enjoying alcohol, gambling and fighting. One day an old monk who practices physiognomy (the study of facial features) met him and directly told him:

"Your face shows the sign of death. You will die within a year if you continue to live the way you live now"

After that warning, Nanboku changed his way of life becoming vegetarian for a year. He became calmer, his facial features changed and supposedly he experienced good fortune in life. Nanboku was attributed with several quotes such as:

"Eating can determine your life"

When we think to the abundance of food choices we have available today in the developed world, we clearly live in a golden period. Our food is safer and more hygienic. We have greater access to meat, fish, vegetables, grains. It tastes good. We have no fear of famine.

Really, our problems are those of excess. We have too much choice and our food portions are too large. We also have other distractions, which indirectly cause overeating. People who eat whilst watching TV or surfing the internet will tend to overeat as their minds are distracted.

The 80% diet is similar in principle to the plan of eating a 'restricted diet'. There have been numerous research studies on the benefits of restricted diets.

For example, in one study – 'Dietary restriction in mice beginning at 1 year of age: effect on life-span and spontaneous cancer incidence, (*Weindruch & Walford. 1982)'*, scientists examined the effects of dietary restriction in middle-aged mice on their life span and risk of cancer.

Middle aged mice, aged 12-13 months old, were fed a restricted diet according to the principle of "undernutrition without malnutrition". A control group was included that were fed a normal amount of food. At the end of the experiment, it was found that the mice on the restricted diet had a 10-20% increase in mean and maximum life survival times and had less incidences of spontaneous lymphoma (a type of blood cancer), indicating that a restricted diet can have a beneficial effect on lifespan and risk of cancer.

In another study - 'A Calory-Restricted Diet Decreases Brain Iron Accumulation and preserves Motor Performance in Old Rhesus Monkeys, (*Eastman et al. 2010*)', a calorie restricted diet was examined for the level of iron accumulation in rhesus monkey brains.

Scientists were already aware that a restricted diet reduces the pathological effects of ageing and extends the lifespan in many species but its effects on the brain was less well known.

This study looked at levels of iron in the brain and found that the group of monkeys with a restricted diet had less levels of iron in some parts of the brain compared to the control group. This is significant because high levels of iron in the brain are related to ageing and are implicated in the development of age related conditions such as Parkinson's and Alzheimer's.

There are numerous other studies to show the benefits of calorie restricted diets. The key thing however is "undernutrition without malnutrition". Food should be nutritious, with adequate levels of proteins, fats and carbohydrates of an amount suitable for your level of activity. You should also include a balance of fibre, vitamins, minerals and antioxidants and if the amount of food is eaten according to the hara hachibu-me rule (eating till only 80% of our stomachs are full), we can potentially slow down our rate of ageing and maybe even protect ourselves from certain types of cancer.

Won't We Starve?

Eating to 80% of our stomach's capacity does not mean that we will under-eat, starve or be consistently hungry. This is not the same as a slim-fast type of diet to lose weight. In fact, there are far more extreme diets, which the human body is capable of following.

For example, in Japan, Ms Michiyo Mori has lived on a diet of only one glass of green vegetable juice per day for the last 15 years. She is the subject of a documentary called 'The Age of No Eating - Eating Light for Love and Compassion' (available on the internet).

At age 21, she was diagnosed with Spinocerebellar Degeneration - a neurological disease where the cranial nerves degenerate and can lead to severe disability. She was given a life expectancy of 5 years. However, she decided to follow a special diet designed by a Dr Koda called the Nishi System of Health Engineering, which incorporated fasting and raw foods. After this improved her health, she gradually reduced her calories down to the point where she could survive on a single glass of green vegetable juice. She outlived her 5-year prognosis and practices as an acupuncturist in Osaka well into her 50's.

I advise that this case is certainly not common and it would be deeply inadvisable for someone to attempt this diet without someone who is an expert in this field to guide them. Serious harm can result. I include the story because it indicates that the human body is capable of much more than we assume it to be.

The quality of what we put in our mouths

The quality and presentation of a meal is just as important as its taste and in many cases, we can tell what kind of food is really good for our body simply by looking, smelling or holding it first. This is mindfulness is action.

For example, if we resist the urge to gobble down a 99 pence hamburger from McDonalds, but instead hold it, look carefully and get a feel for it in our hands.

If we look at the meat and feel the texture of the bread, does it have substance? Does it feel natural or does it feel a little synthetic? If we pull it to pieces and roll it, does it easily turn back into dough? If we handle the meat, how oily is it? Imagine how it would feel if this oil was floating around your blood and lymph vessels. Would it be beneficial or clogging for the body? Smell it and really look at it. Have you ever taken an up and personal close look at it before?

Also consider where this food came from. Think of the factory with men and women dressed in white overalls, hats and face masks operating the machines that churn the dough and push out the rolls. Think about the farms with the cows in pens attached to machines given injections of antibiotics and growth hormones.

The meat is processed, frozen and transported hundreds of miles. I should imagine, there is a significant difference between the original hamburgers produced by McDonalds in the 1950s and the factory conveyer stuff we eat today.

Food and Convalescing Diets

When preparing meals during an illness there is often very little appetite, but if you don't eat something you will get weaker. The problem is that when you eat, you know that that food is going to pass through you causing you diarrhea and discomfort. But, if you don't eat, you will get weaker and your condition can deteriorate.

To address this, meals should be very basic and made up of only one or two ingredients. They should border on being bland. In Chinese and Japanese cuisine, there is a meal called congee.

To put it simply, congee is soft white rice which has been simmered for hours. It is eaten whenever a person is sick or recovering in hospital. To make it more nutritious, an egg can be stirred in. Usually, there are no other ingredients or flavorings although a little salt should be tried to see if it is tolerated. It is a simple soft food designed to take the strain off the digestive system but also to give the body energy.

In Western Europe, porridge oats can also be substituted although it is essential they are very soft. Oats should be soaked in cold water for a few hours before cooking.

Here is the recipe for rice congee:

Congee (Rice Soup)

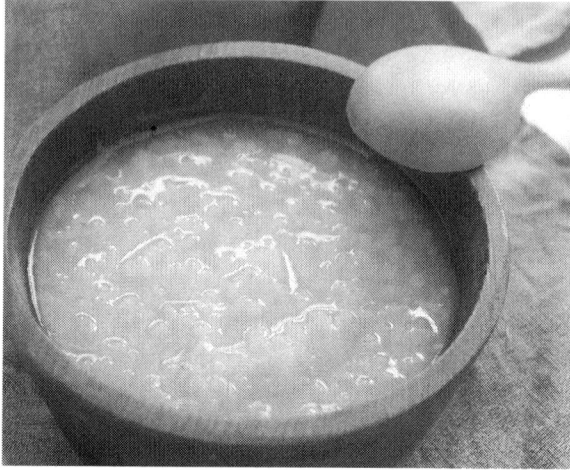

Ingredients:

- ¾ cup long grain rice
- 9 cups water
- 1 teaspoon salt

Preparation:

In a large pot, bring the water and rice to the boil.

When the rice is boiling, turn the heat down to low. Put the lid on the pot, tilting it to allow steam to escape.

Cook on a low heat, stirring occasionally, until the rice has a thick, creamy texture like porridge. Approximately 1-2 hours. Add the salt, taste and add seasonings if desired.

Serve with garnishes. A little soya sauce can be added.

For a healthy option, brown wholegrain rice may be used instead of white rice although the cooking time may have to be increased to 3-4 hours. Alternatively, you can use a pressure cooker and cook for about one hour.

Variations :

For extra nutrition, an egg can be added and stirred into the congee a few minutes before you turn the heat off. Other options are wakame seaweed or nori seaweed, which should be added at the end or kombu seaweed, which should be cooked from the beginning.

A little shredded meat can also be added at the beginning of the cooking process. The long cooking time will mean it is very soft and easy to digest.

Congee tonifys the blood and is very nourishing. It is more easily digestible for the chronically ill person and gentle on the intestines.

Eating when Sick

When we are sick, the digestive system often becomes weaker and less efficient. Digestion requires a lot of energy and so our appetite may reduce so our body can focus on healing. If we are attuned, our bodies will tell us what we can eat and what we cannot. We need simply to listen and obey.

Life sometimes tempts us to ignore these messages. We may be feeling quite run down, overworked, stressed, have a dodgy gut or have the beginnings of a cold or flu, and yet we may still attend that party invitation or that business lunch at a barbecue restaurant and drink alcohol or eat rich oily foods. Later that day, we may get severe stomach cramps and have to rush to A&E with suspected food poisoning. Ignoring these messages can exacerbate or bring on an illness.

Chicken Soup

When your body is a bit stronger and you can tolerate more food, a traditional chicken stew is a way of building up your strength as well as still being relatively easy to digest. It can be suitable for anyone building up their yin energy particularly after a challenging illness, injury or childbirth.

I was told that in Chinese hospitals after childbirth, women are given a highly nutritious broth made of chicken bones simmered for hours, which are designed to rebuild their blood levels and bring a woman's strength back. Women are also kept in hospital for a longer period of time afterwards to recover. Contrast that with NHS hospitals where they will usually discharge you the day after giving birth even with unhealed caesarean scars.

Simple Chicken & Vegetable Stew

Ingredients

3 medium sized potatoes

2 carrots

A few leaves of Chinese cabbage

A handful of spinach

A small slice of ginger

A small spring onion

A small handful of chicken breast meat (free range)

A small handful of brown or white rice.

One organic stock cube (preferably containing no preservatives or additives).

Directions

Peel and chop all the vegetables into small pieces.

Peel the ginger but don't chop it

Chop and slice the chicken into small pieces.

Fill a pan up with water and bring it to the boil. Wash the brown rice, when the water is boiling, put into the pan and stir it. Add the meat and ginger and stir it in. Cook on a low heat for 20 minutes to soften it. Then add the rest of the vegetables. Bring to the boil and simmer for another 30 minutes. Then add the stock cube and stir it in. After cooking, leave to settle and cool.

Serve in a bowl and enjoy a highly nutritious simply cooked soft meal.

White chicken meat is yang and because it has less yang energy than other meats such as lamb or beef, it is easier to digest. It is balanced with yin vegetables. The ginger aids digestion and can help with nausea.

CHAPTER SIXTEEN

RE-ENERGISE WITH MASSAGE & ACUPRESSURE

Receiving a massage can be a deeply relaxing experience and provide many benefits for our bodies. I have worked with many busy professionals as clients who like to include a weekly massage session as part of their health routine to keep themselves in good health. In fact, receiving any kind of massage even if it is from a family member, partner or sometimes even on yourself can provide some benefit.

In the UK, there was a tradition until fairly recently that when a family member is sick, you bring them grapes. I have heard that there is a tradition in India among some people, that when family members are sick, instead you bring oil with you and a younger family members rubs the feet of the sick person. I know which one I would prefer to have.

There are very basic forms of massage that everyone can learn such as basic hand massage or simple acupressure, which they can then give to their own family members or friends if they are sick, but also which you can use on yourself.

For example, whenever we have a headache or shoulder pain, it is common to find our hands drawn to rub our temples or the tops of our shoulders or lower back and sometimes to find a particular point and pressing on it helps relieve tension. This itself is a basic form of acupressure and shows that acupressure is a natural expression of the body guiding us where to press to heal ourselves.

The acupressure points are the same as the acupuncture points as discussed earlier in the section on acupuncture. Acupressure is a basic tool that anyone can learn. In this section, I will go over some basic acupressure points and methods of massaging them. Remember that acupuncture is the technique of manipulating the acupuncture points in order to stimulate a healing response using small needles.

The application of moxibustion, also stimulates these points by using heat from a burning herb. However, it is also possible to stimulate these points using finger pressure, stroking, rubbing or tapping, which is where acupressure comes in.

A few years ago, I attended a talk by an A&E (Accident and Emergency) doctor who had gone on to learn Traditional Chinese Medicine and had written a book. He recounted a story when he applied acupressure to one of his patients with breathing difficulties. He pressed one of the acupuncture points on the person's arm that relates to the 'Lung Channel' and was pleased by the result. This gentle form of acupressure had a beneficial effect on the person's breathing and helped calm the patient.

Self-acupressure can help relieve stress and recharge your energy. Stress in our life causes a tightening of our musculature and a poor flow of Ki. This can cause tiredness because our bodies waste energy by holding onto this tension in the muscles, which could instead be used for other homeostatic functions. Some of this tension can be relieved by acupressure.

We can use the fingers and thumbs to activate these points by either pressing, tapping or massaging these points. These points are all easy to find and touch on ourselves. Acupressure is essentially a meditation. Some of these points can be massaged on family members, or friends also.

Qi / Ki

We discussed earlier about Ki energy and the Channel system, the body's Ki energy is the life force of our body. The Channels are a network where a special kind of Ki travels through the whole body in special pathways – just like a motorway network passes all through the whole of the UK. The Ki travels though these Channels. These Channels are divided in 12 main pathways (actually there are more).

These 12 main pathways travel through various organs in the body and give Ki energy to these organs. Each Channel pathway is named after a particular organ in the body which it travels through and has more influence over. Hence the Stomach Channel pathway travels through the stomach and affects digestion.

Some of these organs are the stomach, spleen, heart, lungs, kidneys and liver. If the Channel is blocked, or if there is not enough Ki, then these organs do not get enough energy. Therefore, we can become tired. If we have a smooth flow of Ki and an adequate amount of Ki, we can be healthy. But if Ki is blocked or is weak in our Channels, we can have health problems.

Acupoints & Acupressure

Along the Channels, there are special openings, which in the West we call acupoints. In Japanese, they are called Tsubo. This is where the Ki of the Channel can be accessed. These points are mapped out and are in the same location on everybody.

When an organ is weak or the Ki is weak, we can stimulate the healing power of the body by treating these acupoints. Treating an acupoint on a specific Channel helps to activate the flow of Ki energy and stimulates the Channel.

Massage Techniques

In Japan and China, they practice different types of massage. In Japan, there is Shiatsu, in China there is Tuina. These words literally translate as 'finger pressure'. Any light gentle pressure is good enough. You do not need to force and strain your hands. Gentle light rotational massage and slight pressure on the points is good enough. Use whichever is comfortable – fingers tips or thumbs. Lightly find the point and slowly increase the pressure and then rotate your thumb or finger. Keep pressing the point.

Namikoshi Shiatsu

Shiatsu, meaning 'finger pressure', is a form of Japanese bodywork. Massage techniques uses finger, thumbs, feet and palms and assisted stretching. Treatments can be carried out on the floor or a treatment couch and involve thumb or finger pressure on a pattern of certain points on the body to relieve pain, help relax and stimulate blood and lymph flow.

Shiatsu evolved from the Chinese massage systems of Tuina and Anma. One of the most influential figures in Shiatsu was Tokujiro Namikoshi who founded a shiatsu college in the 1940s. Since then, shiatsu has grown to be recognized worldwide.

As a young boy, Namikoshi discovered a talent for bodywork. In the early 1900s, his family lived in Hokkaido in the Northern part of Japan - a very cold and harsh area with large amounts of snowfall. The cold weather badly affected his mother who suffered from painful arthritis. As there was no other medical aid available, her children took turns at rubbing her painful joints.

Of all the kids, it was Namikoshi, who's hands helped to relieve her pain the most and so he adopted the role of family physical therapist. His mother told him that it felt better when he pressed on her body rather than stroke or rub, a technique which was to become an essential part of shiatsu therapy.

Namikoshi had the sense in that when he found a cold and stiff point on his mother's body, he would spend more time pressing the point daily until it warmed up and softened. Eventually, with daily shiatsu treatment, his mother's rheumatoid arthritis disappeared.

After this, news of Namikoshi's therapeutic ability spread around the village and his services became in demand. He helped the local school principal's wife start to produce milk again by using his finger pressure technique after it had ceased to flow shortly after the birth of her child. He also travelled with a Buddhist monk and visited local villagers to help them with their health ailments using his skill at locating and treating stiff points.

After formally obtaining his massage license he decided to call his system of massage Shiatsu - a word that he had read in a magazine article, because he felt it closely described the type of therapy he was practicing. He went on to further develop his particular system and help to promote it around the world.

Namikoshi wanted to apply modern scientific understanding of anatomy and physiology to his system. He came to the conclusion that as he pressed certain points on his mother's body, it was like giving natural cortisone shots because he was stimulating her adrenal glands. This led him to believe that the body is able to produce all the chemicals it needs to heal itself, and that all that is needed is to stimulate the body to produce them.

Namikoshi identified that stress had a particularly harmful effect on the body as it causes the body to under-produce or over-produce these chemicals and hormones. He believed that shiatsu has the ability to re-harmonise the body and bring it back into balance and that with shiatsu treatment, it is possible for the person to develop great health and strength as it stimulates the inner healing power.

Namikoshi's abilities spread far and wide. He helped heal a famous Japanese philosopher Ishimaru Gohei, who ended up insuring Namikoshi's fingers for over a hundred thousand yen, the equivalent of about 10 million pounds today. Namikoshi also survived General MacArthur's post war attempts at eradicating 'unscientific' practices in his attempt to modernize the country following Japan's defeat and occupation by the American forces following World War II. According to Saito's account of Namikoshi:

"There were more than 300 unregulated therapies in Japan, and McArthur ordered all to be researched to document which ones had scientific proof of merit and which did not. At the end of eight years, the universities reported back and Shiatsu was the only therapeutic practice that received scientific approval. In 1955, the Japanese Health Ministry legally recognized Shiatsu and it became a licensed therapy".

This is an interesting idea - 'that the body is able to produce all the chemicals it needs to heal itself. In the case of cancer, it is well documented that there are sudden and unexplained cases of spontaneous healing. Usually, when orthodox medicine encounters such a case, they tend to explain it away by saying that the original cancer was misdiagnosed. Yet, it does indicate that the body has some powerful ability to heal itself. The question to be asked is what can bring that effect into being?

Painful Points.

Sometimes when you have stiff shoulders or a headache, you may instinctively rub an area of your shoulders or temples and you may come across a specific point that is especially painful and seems like the source of all the discomfort. In the case of shoulders or back pain, it may be that these points are what physiotherapists call trigger points. If you continue to rub these points, the pain may be relieved. Alternatively, receiving shallow acupuncture needling on these points, can also release them.

In Chinese, such points are called 'Ashi' points - literally *scream aloud* or 'painful' points. They will often be found at key acupuncture point locations. Moxa on these points can also help to relieve the pain. However, if you do not have access to acupuncture treatment, acupressure is a quick and easy way to start working on these points.

If a point on a channel is painful, it indicates that the point is active and that the channel may be affected. These are the best points to use. It means that the energy at this point is more out of balance. Therefore, it needs more care and attention. Massage these points as often as you like or get a family member to do it.

In the next section, we will look at some common acupressure points to practice on yourself or on your family.

To begin: Posture

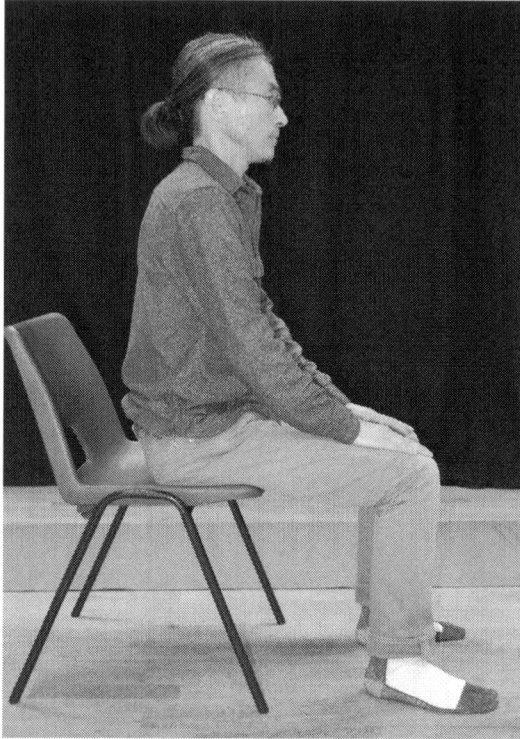

Before commencing self-acupressure, it is a good opportunity to think about your posture and take some deep breaths.

1. Sit up straight, keep the spine straight. This allows energy to flow up and down the spine smoothly.

2. Breathe. Oxygen can really help us with energy, sometimes if we breathe a little shallowly; we don't get enough energy in the body, so if we take a few slow deep breaths it really helps.

3. Breathe in through the nose, hold a few seconds and then breath out through the mouth.

4. If you can, try to breathe deeply into your abdomen. Breathe a few times like this.

5. Loosen the shoulders and chest. Sometimes, tight muscles in the chest and shoulders can restrict breathing. All muscle tension takes away energy. So let's relax these muscles. Do some shoulder rolls, back and then forward, this helps open and relax the chest. Now we have more freedom and energy movement in the chest and torso.

Massage Techniques

There are various techniques that can be used. The key is that whatever massage technique you adopt, it should be comfortable for you and if you are doing it for someone else, it should be comfortable for them.

One method is the Push and Rotate technique. Use your thumbs and sink them into the acupressure point. Then gradually rotate your thumb and massage the point. Do it gently and gradually increasing the pressure if needed. Feel yourself melt into the point, rather than just force your thumb in clumsily. If you feel pain, ease off.

If you are treating someone else, be careful not to be too gung-ho or to try to show off your strength by pushing too hard. This is the ego acting. Also don't assume that 'no pain no gain' is the right approach. People with Yin type bodies may find it too uncomfortable. Always communicate and make sure the person is fine with the pressure.

In some types of Chinese and Thai massage, painful and strong pressure massage is common and can help to move things quickly. These types of massage are more Yang in nature and can leave a person feeling sore afterwards. For the purposes of this book, we will focus on gentler (more Yin) types of techniques.

Pictures—Push & Rotate

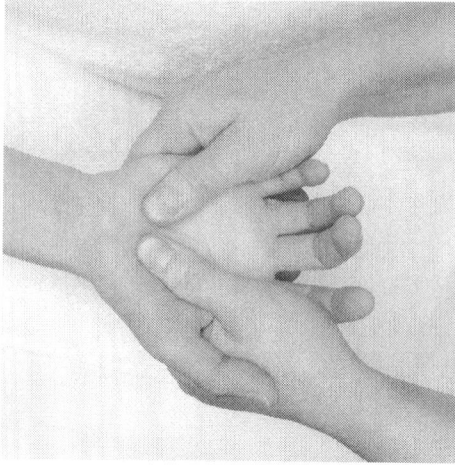

Techniques: Tapping

Tapping is another gentle technique which is also incorporated as part of Emotional Freedom Technique (EFT). It is quite simply tapping on the acupuncture points with the fingers, hands or gently with the knuckles. Tapping is a more Yin technique.

Common Acupressure Points to invigorate the Body and help with tiredness:

Large Intestine 4 – Hegu / Gokoku

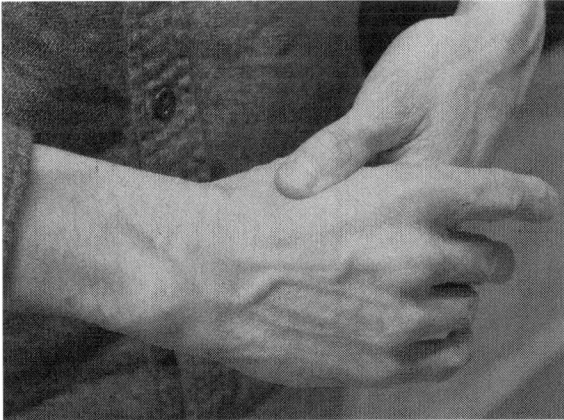

This is a commonly used point with many different actions. It can help with strengthening the general constitution, pain relief, constipation and toothache.

It is not usually advisable to massage this acupressure/acupuncture point in pregnant women as it has a downward stimulating effect on the Ki energy in the body.

Pericardium 8 – Laogong / Rokyu

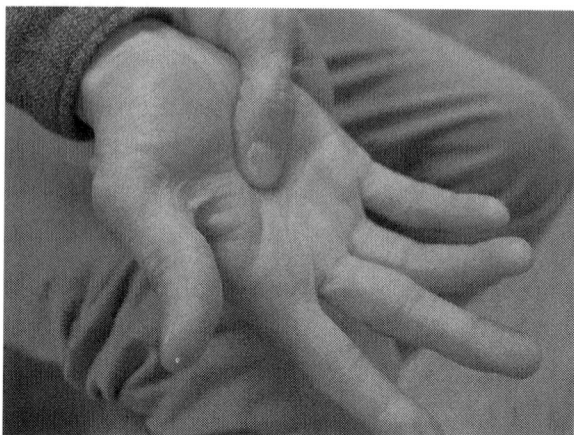

Taoist practitioners and other energy-healers frequently use the palms of their hands as a place from which to emit energy. The Chinese name for this point is Lao Gong. "Gong" means palace, and "Lao" means labor or toil.

This point has a stimulating effect on our own bodymind. It helps calm the spirit and resolving fatigue. If you are feeling anxious, it is an easy point to massage in any situation.

Du 20 - Bahui / Hyaku-e

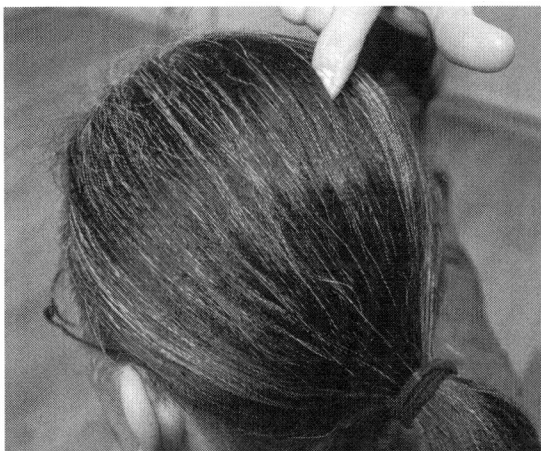

Put your fingers behind both your ears on either side of your head and then move them upwards to the top of the scalp until they meet in the middle. Then in that area, feel around for a small indentation. When you find that indentation, you have the point. Make sure you are on the midline. You can find the midline by marking it at the point between your eyebrows

This point is called Bahui in Chinese. It is the meeting point of many energy channels in the body. It brings your energy up. If we activate the point, we can also raise our mental awareness

You can lightly tap the point or massage it, or do both. Do so for a few seconds to activate the point.

Prenatal and Post Natal Ki-Energy

Our energy levels can be related to two types of energies in the body: Prenatal and Post-natal energy.

Prenatal Energy

Pre-natal energy is the energy we are born with. It is the fundamental life force that we are supplied with from our ancestors – the energy that takes us through the various periods of growth and changes of life.

We are born with an abundance of it at birth. As we grow older, we gradually use it up. It is also an energy that is important for helping us recover from health problems.

This pre-natal energy is related to the Kidney organ and the Kidney Channel. Therefore, we use these acupressure points to stimulate our prenatal energy and give it a boost.

Acupuncture point to stimulate prenatal energy:

Kidney 27 - Shu Fu / Yu-fu

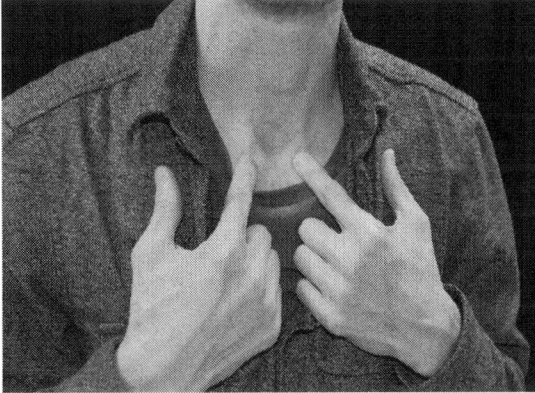

These two points, on both sides of the chest, are close to your sternum and just below the collarbone.

Tap these points - either with one hand – one at a time or with both hands at the same time. You can tap with the fingers or the hands or light fist. It's fine if you don't find the exact point – as long as you are in the right area. You can also press and rub these points to stimulate them.

These points are used by the famous hypnotist – Paul McKenna to help give up addictions. These points also help to awaken your energy. Tarzan used to bang on these points when he yelled out. Maybe he did this because it gave him energy.

Location: In a depression on the lower border of the clavicle, 2 inches lateral to the midline. Feel for the tender area just under the clavicle bone and massage gently.

Action : Improves Kidney deficiency and adrenal exhaustion - improves fatigue.

Post Natal Energy

This is the energy that we gain externally from the universe. It is the energy that we get from food and drink and from breathing. As we all know, we eat regularly and drink water to replenish our energy. We build our bodies from the protein, our energy comes from carbohydrates. Fibre provides us with some vitamins and minerals and helps our digestive health.

But more importantly then eating good food is our ability to absorb. If our digestive system is weak, we cannot convert the food effectively into energy and we can become tired.

In Traditional Oriental medicine, it is the Spleen and Stomach organ and Channel that is related to the digestive system, which is responsible for converting substances we consume into energy. Therefore, we massage points on these Channels to stimulate these organs.

Acupressure points to stimulate postnatal energy:

Stomach 36 – Zusanli / Ashi san li

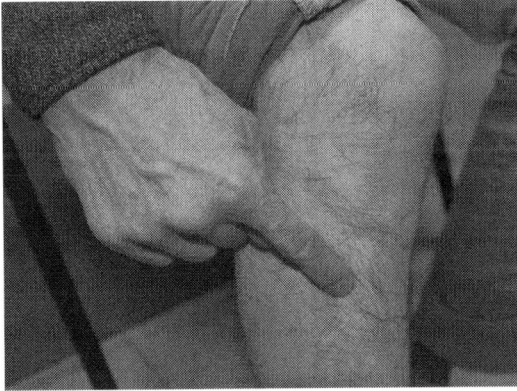

The English translation of this point is "Leg Three Mile" - meaning that if we stimulate this point we will have the power to walk an extra 3 miles.

Location:

Below the knee, on the outer part of the leg, approximately three finger breaths down from the knee cap and one finger breath to the side of the tibia bone. Rest your hands on the side of your kneecaps and feel for the tender or tight area and massage.

Actions: General Weakness

Finally, self-acupressure can also be incorporated into a small daily health practice taking 10 to 15 minutes starting with the warm up stretches and breathing, followed by the acupressure and then ending with a warm down. A helpful warm down can include exercises to balance the fire and water energy of our body.

Fire below, water above

In the modern world, we use our brains too much. We think or worry too much. We use our eyes excessively looking at our smartphones or TV. It means that all the energy is in our head. But in Traditional Oriental Medicine, it is important to not use the head too much but to keep our energy in the lower belly where many of our important organs are.

One of the themes in this book is that of *fire below and water above*, which can also be described as *keep a warm belly and a cool head*. The lower belly is called the dantian (hara) in Japanese. In Oriental medicine and martial arts, the lower belly is said to be the powerhouse of the body. It is the source of our power.

When you feel tired, if you do not feel like massaging these acupuncture points, simply lay your hands on your lower belly, below the naval, one hand on top the other and breathe slowly and deeply.

As you breathe in, watch your hands slightly rise. As you breathe out, your hands sink down. This brings the energy away from your head and puts it back into the power center of your body so that you can conserve your energy and recharge. It is also incredibly relaxing.

Power Centre Meditation: Laying on of hands

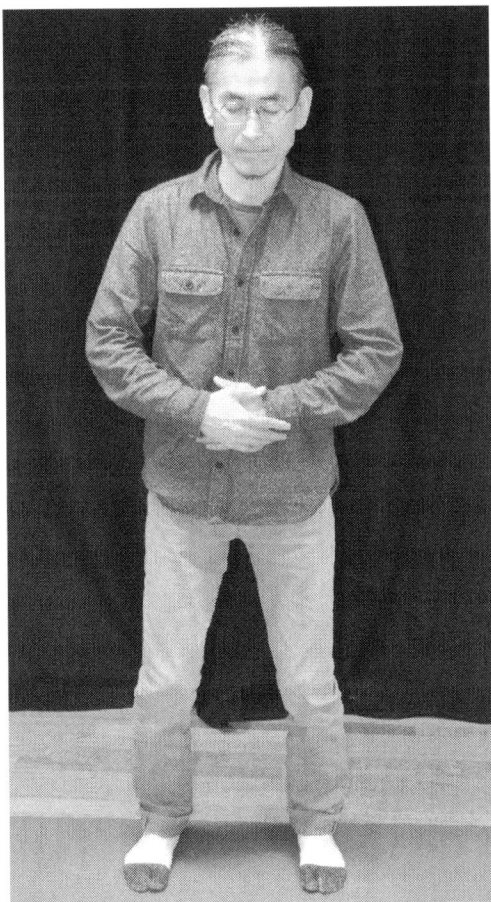

Simply lay your hands on your lower belly and breathe or make a gentle circular motion with your hands in a clockwise direction. Do this for 3-5 minutes or longer if possible.

Warm Down: Face rub

Finally, after your short meditation - laying on of hands, it is time to quickly awaken yourself again ready to face the world with the face rub.

Rub the hands together as fast as you are able. Then place the hands over your face and hold over your eyes. Hold here for a few seconds and then rub your face gently. Rub again and repeat. You will feel your face relax.

This is a way to make ourselves more alert. We hold a lot of tension in our face muscles especially if we are upset, angry annoyed and this tension makes us tired. By rubbing our face, we relax these muscles, and bring energy to our eyes and head.

By rubbing the hands together, it brings energy and warmth into your hands. Then when you touch your face, it brings that same warmth and energy to your face. Even if you rub slowly - there is a positive effect.

All of these steps together will improve the energy in your body, will relax you and also help increase your energy. If you breathe well, eat well, relax and tap or massage these points - all these little things together will have a positive effect on your body.

CHAPTER SEVENTEEN

RELATIONSHIPS AND OUR PLACE IN SOCIETY

和

Wa - 'Harmony'

A source of tension is our relationships with others. Marital disharmony, or a break with our parents, bullying co-workers or boss, anti-social neighbors playing music loud at night or acting in an intimidating manner all create stress for us.

The most extreme is when society completely breaks down with mugging and burglary common, or at the most extreme, a civil war as we have seen in some Middle Eastern or North African countries in recent years. Stress at the national level, creates stress at the local community level, then at the family level and in each and every one of us. The family is simply the smallest unit of the state.

If we have harmony in ourselves, we contribute to a harmonious family life. If the family is harmonious, it contributes to a harmonious community. If the community is harmonious, neighbors have good relationships, and each household is concerned about keeping their area clean of rubbish and well maintained and participate in local community meetings and celebrations.

It ensures the larger community is orderly with local services running efficiently like the fire service, ambulances, schools, waste disposal, and creates a productive atmosphere where local businesses and shops can flourish creating wealth for all to benefit from.

This is the concept of 和 (wa) in Japanese, which means harmony and is a concept that underpins all of Japanese society. It is the reason why service is Japan is seen as exceptional and public expressions of anger are looked down on. It is one of the reasons why Japan has one of the most efficient societies and strongest economies in the world.

Confucianism

Japan, China and Korea are relatively collectivist societies where harmony and relationships between people are placed more importantly that the rights of the individual, regardless of how they may impact on others around them. In Japan, the concept of 'Wa' or harmony, particular in maintaining harmony between yourself and others is seen as especially important.

Another aspect of harmony and order is that of respect for hierarchy, respect for the family and respect for the community.

One of the philosophies that has influenced the development of these types of societies is *Confucianism*, a philosophy of life based on the teachings of Confucius.

Confucius was a Chinese philosopher who lived around 552BC to 479BC. He travelled throughout China with a small group of disciples. His group underwent many hardships in their travels in order to spread his teachings designed to improve the society they lived in.

Confucianism is not so much a religion as a set of ethical principles that emphasis respect for the family, the elders, societal obligations and rules of courtesy particularly between rulers and subject, community members, husband and wife and between parents and children. Some key concepts are the adherence of rituals, virtuous example, self-cultivation, gentlemanly behaviour and becoming a learned man.

I have summarized some of Confucius's teachings taken from the book of his teaching, The Analects:

On daily self-improvement:

"Zengzi said, every day I examine myself on three points: When I worked to benefit someone else, did I do my best? In my relationships with my friends, did I fail to be trustworthy? Did I pass on any knowledge I myself had not put into practice?"

On gentlemanly behaviour:

"There are nine things the gentleman gives thought to: he aims to be clear in vision, keen in hearing, amicable in his expression, courteous in his manners, conscientious in carrying out his words, and respectful in attending to his responsibilities; and when he is in doubt, he asks questions; when he is angry, he reflects on the unwanted consequences this could cause; when he sees a chance for gain, he asks whether it is right".

"A gentleman does not try to stuff himself when he eats and is not worried about the comfort of his dwelling. He is anxious about getting things done and careful about what he says. He gravitates towards those who possess moral integrity because he wants to put himself right. One could say that he is someone who loves learning".

On relationship between the parent and child:

"A youngster should be filial to his parents when he is at home and respectful to his elders when he is away from his home. He should be prudent in action and trustworthy in words".

On learning:

"The gentleman makes plans to realize the *Way*; he does not make plans to secure food. If you decide to till the field, there will still be time when you go hungry. If you decide to devote yourself to learning, there will be times when you may receive an official stipend (for putting your knowledge to work). The Gentleman worries about the *Way*. He does not worry about being poor"

There are some common themes that come up in these quotes. One is the importance on emphasizing internal personal qualities like integrity, work, knowledge and manners.

In our current age, there has been a great emphasis on material gains – wardrobes full of clothes, new cars bought on credit, the buying of houses, which has led to property bubbles and unaffordable housing throughout the Western world, rich food, which has led to obesity and poor health, even money, which has led to one of the greatest economic crashes in the last one hundred years.

In a way, it could be said we have focused too much on the yang (external wants and possessions) and neglected the yin (internal qualities and our internal state). We do need a certain degree of security and comfort. Our basic needs must be met, but we mustn't forget to consider the development of our internal qualities.

I remember a story my father told me from when he was younger. Being of the post war generation, he had a very limited education and was working full time in manual labour jobs as soon as he left school. However, he was not proud of his lack of education and grew very tired of the types of conversations he would have to listen to from his co-workers which focused almost entirely on *"Tits, bums and horses"* or in other words, woman and gambling.

He chose to go to night school whilst working to pick up his 'O' levels and eventually went to university as a mature student. After he obtained his degree, he had a short stint working in offices and in teaching but soon returned to manual labour working, which he preferred.

The point of getting the degree was never to improve his income or status. It was simply to improve himself. The message from Confucius is that the path to being a gentleman comes not from status or the outward show of wealth but from learning and self-improvement. I believe that even a poor man, wearing the humblest of clothes can be a true gentleman as it is based on his values, his integrity and his actions.

Respect for the society we live in

Respect for society, the community and for our elders must be cultivated at an early age, otherwise, there is a risk that selfish behavior may take hold. Discipline and firm boundaries are a part of this.

In short, Confucianism is about respect for the family, for society, and contributing and becoming a useful member. It works both ways. Adults must respect children and guide them wisely into adulthood as well as setting firm boundaries. Children must respect their elders and learn discipline, the meaning of work and of contributing to society.

Of course, this is not always the case. There are situations when parents can be a wholly negative influence on the family and in these situations it is necessary for children to protect and distance themselves. Also, there comes a time when children must break from their parents and find their own way in life.

The principles of Confucianism underpin all traditional stable societies. Whenever a society breaks against tradition that holds its society together, it risks anarchy and collapse. We see this in my country the UK.

For example, a common pastime is football. One of the UK's greatest exports is football hooliganism. In the past, whenever the national team went abroad, a legion of fans followed with the express purpose of excessive drinking, violence and destroying of property.

Things have improved now, but British football supporters still have the worst reputation in Europe. Spanish and Greek holiday resorts are well aware of the wild and alcoholic tendencies of their British holidaymaker *guests*. Yet it was not always so.

The famous English Novelist George Orwell observed in 1944:

"An imaginary foreign observer would certainly be struck by our gentleness; by the orderly behaviour of English crowds, the lack of pushing and quarrelling...and except for certain well-defined areas in half a dozen big towns, there is very little crime or violence".

In my own country, these changes in the national psyche and attitudes have occurred over the last few decades. The cause is simply an increase in selfishness and a lack of consideration for others.

In comparison, why are Japanese tenants often favoured by landlords? Why do hotels often favour Japanese tourists? Are they some kind of superhuman or gifted race? Of course not, they are no different from anyone else, but it is their attitudes that have given them a favoured reputation.

The Japanese are widely perceived to be polite, well behaved and respectful of other cultures when abroad. One of the reasons for this attitude can be found in this Japanese saying:

迷惑をかけない

Meiwaku o kakenai

Cause no trouble

'Cause no trouble' is an important rule in Japanese society. This expression can be described as 'being considerate of others'. An example of this can be found in the story of George Ohsawa, the founder of Macrobiotics (a Japanese healthy living lifestyle plan):

> "When he was a toddler, he (Ohsawa) was playing one day throwing pieces of coal into a rain puddle. The water splashed and dirtied the side of the neighbour's house.
>
> This act violated the cardinal rule of 'Meiwaku O Kakenai' - consideration for others and his mother struck him so hard that blood ran freely from his nose. She then tied him up with cord until his father came home to repeat the beating".

That something as simple as splashing dirty water onto the side of someone's house is seen worthy of a severe punishment, reflects the importance of consideration for others in Japan in the early part of the 20th century. Yet today, far worse behaviours are tolerated by parents today even when they clearly cause annoyance to others.

I lived in Japan a short time and was struck by some significant differences between people and communities between Japan and my home country the UK.

Firstly, there was generally less anti-social behavior in public places. Anyone who has walked past a small group of teenagers hanging around outside a local off-licence or convenience store in the UK has to prepare themselves to receive any number of rude remarks, insults or requests to buy alcohol or cigarettes for these *children*.

Any kind of anti-social behavior that is witnessed such as graffiti, dropping litter, feet on chairs in trains or buses, loudness or general rude intimidating behaviour in a public place tends to be ignored. This is because any kind of confrontation with the offenders can result - at best in being sworn at, or worst actual physical violence.

I never saw anything like this in Japan. Consequently, there is more trust. There are vending machines in even very remote areas of Japan which sell soft drinks, beer (yes - beer) and cigarettes. These machines remain undamaged and intact.

In the UK, these machines would probably last at best one night before they were broken into or had graffiti sprayed all over them. Driving on Japanese roads, there is less of the impatience of other drivers with aggressive tailgating or overtaking who are in a rush and significantly less outbursts of anger. The community is more cohesive.

Litter can be seen as a barometer of a society. Where there is lots of detritus, we can assume we see a less cohesive society, with less respect for the surroundings and the community. One time at a local train station in Yokohama, I saw a group of school kids instructed to go there and pick up rubbish. I watched them in their school uniforms diligently picking up rubbish.

In fact, in all of Japan, you will be hard pressed to find rubbish on the street. In the UK, I regularly see school kids at hometime, dropping litter - empty packets of crisps and chocolate bag wrappers. Perhaps many of us are unaware that this has become the norm, when it fact it is something completely abnormal and actually reflects a dis-harmonious society.

Ceremony in Daily Life

Ceremony may seem like a pointless exercise, with no significant meanings or carry with it a throwback to times when we were more superstitious and hence more primitive. However, the following of ceremony, even small insignificant one's help create a bond between the people of a society. It is these bonds that create a coherency, trust and loyalty to your country and your fellow countrymen as well as to uphold the traditions of the society.

In Japan, there are many different traditional ceremonies for all stages of life and development which are taken seriously. For children, there are the coming of age ceremonies of girls and boys, which are carried out separately. These are traditional ceremonies participated by the whole family where kimonos (traditional outfits) are worn.

For newborns, there is a ceremony called Okuizome, held 100 days after a baby's birth in which the infant is imitatively fed with solid foods such as fish, rice and specially prepared vegetables in a ceremony to signify that the child will never go without food for the rest of his or her life.

At this age, the child is not able to eat solids yet, so usually, one of the oldest members of the household holds the baby and touches the food to the baby's mouth with chopsticks. The food also has to be given to the baby in a very specific order.

Another ceremony, similar to the Western baptism, is called Miyamairi. It is where a newborn baby is taken to a shrine one month after their birth for a special ceremony to prey for his or her health and happiness. In this ceremony, the baby wears a special cloth.

These are just a few examples, but Japanese culture is full of many types of ceremonies for all stages of life, coming of age, death and following death. Perhaps they seem tedious, but they do ensure that family and extended family will have many opportunities to meet and maintain their connections.

As Japan has adopted modern consumerist and corporate lifestyles it stills holds dearly its past traditions to counterbalance the excesses and materialist type nature of the modern world. Many of these ceremonies involve the family which helps keep bonds and connections strong.

Respect for the family

In the UK, the traditional family has been weakened and its various roles replaced by the state, which has attempted to become like a surrogate family. We see this in the increase in divorces, single parent families, the complete outsourcing of education, health and care of the elderly to the state and the replacement of the family roles and responsibilities with the welfare state.

Another importance of strong ties comes in the treatment and care of elderly family members. In Japan, the tradition is that parents are cared for by the son's new family. Though it can be very demanding dealing with an elderly parent or grandparent who may be suffering from dementia or incontinence, this is part of the social contract that binds families.

In the West, the issue is not so straightforward and can be a source of stress and guilt. We may not have the capacity financially or physically to look after our parents and will rely on the outsourcing of care. Also, if our parents have lived a life of self-interest, putting their own wants ahead of the family, then our obligation to care for them as they reach old age is reduced and perhaps we don't see why we should look after them now.

Whether elderly relatives are put in home or we care for them is something that we must decide according to our own personal circumstances, however, we must be aware that our own kids will watch how we deal with our parents and learn from our example.

Sometime in the future, our care will be in their hands. This is the importance of family obligations and maintaining good relations between the generations. This expression, which is sometimes used as a joke has truth in it: 'Be nice to your children, for they will choose your nursing home'.

CHAPTER EIGHTEEN

DEALING WITH LIFE'S CHALLENGES

猿も木から落ちる

Saru mo ki kara ochiru

Even monkeys fall out of the tree.

This well-known Japanese proverb – 'even monkeys fall out of the tree', implies that anyone can fail at some point in their life. In fact, it is our failures that define our human existence.

Perhaps the most interesting people we come across are those that have faced and dealt with adversity. Unfortunately, failure can be a painful and potentially destructive experience. A little failure can make us stronger. But if we have too much, it can bring on stress, tension, negative emotions and lead to sickness, sometimes even death.

Failure and guilt seem to go together. When we fail – whether it is an exam, a relationship, a duty, a job interview, a loss of a loved one, or a loss of a job, a sport, or if part of our body becomes sick, this supposed 'failure' can be devastating to our psyche and can bring with it feelings of guilt, remorse, blame and inferiority.

Suffice to say, in the short term, this is a natural response, which hopefully passes and we can move on with our lives. If we can learn from these experiences – more so the better because failure brings with it a gift – the gift of wisdom. It is the person who never fails who may be the dullest person you will ever speak to at a party.

Fortunately (or *unfortunately*), most of us will have failed at some point in our lives at something. Because failure is an intrinsic part of life. It teaches us to be humbler, to learn to accept that things are not always going to go well. Humans tend by their nature to seek a life of equilibrium, a life without too many ups and downs.

Even a life with too many ups has the potential to unbalance us. We see this in the life of celebrities. Too many lows lead to depression, helplessness and suicidal thoughts. The few ups in life are a cause of gratitude and celebration, the downs – we hope to be able to deal with when they happen without being too distraught. For life has both.

On a national level, perhaps no country has failed as extremely as Japan. From its modernization during the Meiji period and success in the First World War it became a strong country with an international standing.

Following its defeat in the second world war, the country was left devastated - its major cities destroyed, its people starving and demoralized. Occupied by a foreign power. Its international reputation in tatters.

However, its people had a strong work ethic, spirit and determination with a preparation to work hard for the better of the country. 50 years after the end of the war, Japan had the 2nd biggest economy in the world. It led the world in the manufacture of electronics, motorcycles and in the car industries. Their car industry even surpassed that of Ford.

One of the reasons for Japanese success is the concept of 'Kaizen' - meaning 'change for the better' which can be interpreted as making daily improvements to become more efficient and eliminate what does not work. It is a philosophy that has led to Japanese technology being synonymous with high quality and value for money.

Kaizen is a concept that we can apply to our own health and lives. The exercises and health practices in this book can be part of a daily kaizen practice. If every day, we make small incremental improvements to our breathing habits or spend a few minutes stretching or using our bodies more, we can make 'change for the better'. Small daily improvements can set a good direction for our life no matter what situation we are in.

Some people believe that we are only given the level of problems in life that we are able to deal with, to test us, to make our spirit grow. Against a background of having our fundamental needs met, that may be true. A family living in a third world shanty town without running water or electricity or a refugee escaping a war-torn country might disagree.

Fundamentally, failures or struggles in life make us tough. Life is tough. There are joys and wonderful things, but there are struggles and knock-downs. Sometimes, we can deal with them. Sometimes not.

There is another Japanese proverb:

雨降って地固まる

Ame futte ji katamaru

The rain falls, the ground hardens

'The rain falls, the ground hardens' implies an uncomfortable situation, but one that makes us firmer and stronger either physically, mentally or spiritually, depending on the nature of the difficulty.

These challenges also make us humble and teach us to re-evaluate our lives and priorities. Failure is as much a part of life as success. Failure teaches our souls many lessons that we cannot learn from experiencing only success alone, (or what we consider to be success in life).

When failure comes, our challenge is to face it with grace and acceptance. To not get angry, resentful or blame others. Disaster is always one step away from us at any point in life. It is our shadow. Perhaps the best approach is to adopt a playful attitude. We can take example from the American karate fighter, Williams, as he talks to the evil Mr Han in the Bruce Lee movie, Enter the Dragon:

Enter the Dragon

Mr Han: - "We are all ready to win, just as we are born knowing only life. It is defeat that you must learn to prepare for."

Williams: - "I don't waste my time with it. When it comes, I won't even notice."

Mr Han: - "Oh. How so?"

Williams: - "I'll be too busy looking good."

CHAPTER NINETEEN

IKIGAI – LIFE SATISFACTION

生きがい

Ikigai

Satisfaction and Purpose in Life

In Japan, the word ikigai relates to life satisfaction, self-esteem, morale, happiness as well as an evaluation of the meaning of one's own life and usefulness.

This concept has particularly been studied among the aged in Japan, which has had one of the largest increases in the proportion of people aged 65 and over in the world - a figure around 25% of the population in 2015. With such an ageing society, the issue of health - both physical and mental is of considerable importance.

In one study on ikigai, over 4000 elderly members of the Silver Human Resources Center (SHRC), a public temporary employment agency, were given questionnaires to study their level of ikigai. To give an example of how ikigai was assessed, one of the questions asked was: "Do you want to work in the community to use what you have learned and experienced to make a contribution to society?".

The fact that Japan has an employment agency set up specifically for the elderly puts it well ahead of other western countries, where the moment you reach retirement age, people feel they are put out to pasture.

The SHRC is a vocational placement agency for people providing work to those over the age of 60 years old throughout Japan, and is supported by the national and local governments and operates with one of the purposes of enhancing ikigai by providing job opportunities as a social activity not merely as an economic activity. For example: -

My in-laws who live in a small rural town needed some work done to replace the flooring in one of the rooms in their house. They contacted the local Silver Centre and were able to get the work done inexpensively and to a very high standard by its members who had previously worked in the industry.

Factors that raise ikigai

For men, some of the answers that indicated a good level of ikigai, was having a healthy life score (being in relatively good health), being active with work at the SHRC, as well as satisfaction with their life history. The number of rooms in their residence and annual income was also associated with ikigai.

For women, factors that indicated a higher level of ikigai were the presence of a spouse as well as a degree of satisfaction with their life history.

In general, for men, ikigai depended on their work, contribution and health condition, as well as socio-economic factors such as annual income and size of residence. For women, family relations such as a spouse and psychological factor like satisfaction with one's life history were important.

Essentially, ikigai is about being satisfied with your life, finding a place in society and having control of one's life. It is a deeper concept than simply having plenty of possessions or status. It is about what makes us feel true satisfaction with our life at whatever stage of it we are in.

We would all do well to ask of ourselves what would give me ikigai? Is it better family relationships, fulfilling work, contributing to society in some particular way. It is my belief that it is never too late or early to focus on ikigai, as we see in the example of the senior Citizens of the Japanese Silver Resource center who took part in this study. To give another example,

When I lived in Yokohama, a prefecture south of Tokyo which has a relatively large foreign population, I used to attend a local community center where I would get free or very lowly priced Japanese lessons given by ex-Japanese teachers and other retirees.

These wonderful people organized a professional syllabus and lesson calendar . They also ran annual festivals and other activities to help the local foreigners to adapt to the country, learn Japanese and to provide value to the community.

These people were contributing to creating a cohesive society, by volunteering their time, skill and expertise to help a disjointed foreign expat community come together and become part of the local community and I am truly grateful for the time I spent with them. In this way, they obtained a level of ikigai. And I got to be a small part of the community.

Even in the UK, it is possible to contribute to enhance the community. I volunteered and then took a paid position for a few years at St Joseph's hospice in East London. Most hospices are in the charity sector.

At this hospice and at hospices around the country, they are always seeking volunteers from any background, nationality or age to contribute in any way possible, whether it is spending a few hours working in a tea bar, doing filing and admin work, cutting hair, gardening, driving patients to appointments, doing manicures, reading to people on the wards, supporting groups, running meditation classes, complementary therapies or any number of other roles. I have yet to meet anyone, who has not realized a greater level of life satisfaction by contributing some of their time to this purpose.

Without wanting to end this chapter on a low note, the researchers in Japan, found that lower levels of ikigai were associated with a higher risk of death and less healthy ageing in the later stages of life.

Ultimately ikigai relates to the emotions and what gives a person life satisfaction. These researchers focused on elderly members who were relatively fit and who were willing to work for the SHRC. It was hypothesized that the level of ikigai is enhanced among those engaging in productive activities after retirement age and can contribute to a healthier level of ageing.

Choose your retirement age

The retirement age of 65 is an arbitrary figure but does not necessarily mean a person is 'past it'. They may have many years of productive activity left in them. It is those that retire and expect to spend their retirement years in a Spanish villa, on cruises, or playing golf, who may discover that their increased leisure time is not as enjoyable as they thought it would be.

My father is in in his late 70s and still works a manual job as a gardener. It is my belief that his continued work keeps him fit. Mentally he still feels young. My father-in-law, is also past retirement age. He occasionally works part-time and keeps himself continually occupied with working on his electronics, doing housework or driving around. He too is fit and able. Ageing is both a mental and physical thing.

There are plenty of opportunities to enhance ikigai at any stage or age of life and for a healthier state of mind it would be prudent to do so. The concept of ikigai appears to be tied with having good relationships with others, opportunities to communicate with others and providing service to the community either by work or voluntary activities.

•

CHAPTER TWENTY

BACKGROUND OF TRADITIONAL ORIENTAL MEDICINE

The Growing Popularity of Traditional Oriental Medicine

Today, an increasing number of people are experiencing Traditional Oriental Medicine such as Acupuncture, Shiatsu or Chinese massage or are taking herbal remedies. The self-defense arts such as Karate and Kung-Fu are practiced worldwide by millions, helped primarily with the impact of Bruce Lee in the 1970s, but it is also the 'soft' health preservation arts like Tai Chi and Qi gong which have increased in popularity.

Lifestyle magazines often have articles on various celebrities undergoing Facial Acupuncture or Cupping to improve their health or their appearance. We see images of the actress Gwyneth Paltrow and Olympic Gold Medalist swimmer Michael Phelps with round bruises on their bodies from the practice of suction cupping. Often, lifestyle magazines may run articles talking about the benefits of various complementary therapies such as acupuncture for infertility. It is not just the well-off that have access to these therapies.

This popularity has extended into the medical system. In several countries - the US, Australia and several European states, these therapies are covered under medical insurance.

In my own county - the UK, acupuncture is available on the National Health Service (NHS). Along with the more traditional 'classically' trained acupuncturists like myself who have longer training, doctors, nurses and physiotherapists are also able to undergo short courses to learn acupuncture techniques.

In 2001, all Complementary and Alternative Medicine (CAM) therapies were put under the spotlight by the House of Lords in a special report, which found that overall Complementary Therapies are safe and that there is a growing demand for them.

Some of the reasoning to its popularity was that these kinds of therapies led to greater patient satisfaction due to the longer time spent in consultation and treatment. When you contrast that with the average time of five minutes for a consultation with a Medical General Practitioner along with the long waiting lists for an NHS hospital appointment, it is not difficult to see where this satisfaction comes from.

Since this report, CAM therapies have continued to grow in popularity and usage among the general population. Therapies like acupuncture, reflexology, and aromatherapy have become more regulated and their use more integrated into mainstream medicine.

There are even two NHS Complementary Medicine hospitals in the UK - the Royal Hospital for Integrated Health, which offers homeopathy, acupuncture, herbal medicine and other complementary therapies and the NHS Gateway clinic in Lambeth, London which offers acupuncture, herbal medicine and qigong.

Its use in hospices is also growing. For example, at the time of writing, St Joseph's Hospice in East London, where I worked for a few years as an acupuncturist has one of the largest Complementary Therapies Department in the country.

The qualification of acupuncture and herbal medicine, which is now at a degree level BSc level has become a recognized occupation, with acupuncture and Chinese herbal medicine degree courses available to study in Universities throughout Europe and an increasing number of people training in these fields.

I find that less people are generally surprised nowadays when I get asked that standard question 'what do you do?' In fact, people often tell me, 'Oh yes, I had acupuncture once - for such and such problem'.

What kind of people go for Oriental medicine?

Traditional Chinese Medicine is and should always be accessible to all. In China, it is part of the state system of medicine and its treatments are available at a very low cost alongside modern medical treatment.

In Japan and Western countries, it is primarily a therapy that is paid for privately and prices can be more than many people are prepared to pay, which is a shame, but with the increasing number of qualified practitioners in the West, this is changing and more lower cost options are becoming available such as community or multi-bed acupuncture clinics.

The beauty of traditional medicine is that anyone can benefit from it regardless of background, income level or belief system. Though, there have been a few high-profile celebrities that have used Traditional Oriental Medicine such as Madonna, Cher, Sean Connery, Mariah Carey and even Sarah Michel Gellers dog (undergoing animal acupuncture), it is not just for the wealthy.

As an acupuncturist practicing in London in the UK, I am fortunate to have encountered patients from various backgrounds from the student wanting to reduce stress, the housewife with painful periods, people overcoming drug dependency, the London Cockney in his 70's dealing with cancer, the bricklayer with a bad back and the city worker with stiff shoulders and back pain.

The versatility and flexibility of Traditional Oriental Medicine means that it is able to offer some help or relief to all of these people and many more.

Types of Traditional Oriental Medicine

There are several branches to what comprises Traditional Oriental Medicine. Massage, which is known as "tuina" in China or "shiatsu" or "amma" in Japan are types of massage which employ finger or thumb pressure, rolling, and strokes, which tend to be firmer than the gentler effleurage techniques of Swedish massage and can be used for general relaxation as well as to deal with specific complaints.

Another component is herbal medicine which involves pre-prepared pills or formulas or small paper bags containing carefully selected herbs and roots and other substances to be boiled at home.

Most people today are familiar with acupuncture. Acupuncture is the insertion or surface-contact of needles of various sizes and construction onto specific points on the body known as acupuncture points in order to bring about a beneficial reaction.

An adjunct to acupuncture also exists known as moxibustion which is where a processed herb, mogwort (*Artemius vulgaris*) is burnt directly on or indirectly on the acupuncture points or regions of the body. There are various versions of moxibustion e.g. a cigar shaped tube which can be held over the points and small cones that can be placed on the acupuncture points and burnt.

Also, moxa can be rolled into small rice grain sized pieces or threads and burnt on these points. Moxa can also be placed on the end of needles to send heat deeper into the acupuncture points through the needles. There are also smokeless versions of moxa. Some therapists such as Ms. Koshishi in Tokyo only practice moxibustion therapy and never use needles. There is also a system of Moxa therapy called the Sawada system in Japan.

Traditional Oriental Medicine can also be considered as comprising the physical and spiritual health practices such as Qigong – sometimes described as a form of Chinese yoga, Tai Chi – a set of gentle exercises based on the repetition of patterns of movements and which also has a martial arts component, and Meditation, which according to some sources, may potentially lead to the curing of diseases.

Traditional medicine also encompasses dietary therapy – the eating of foods according to the principles of yin and yang and in accordance with nature. It could be argued that Macrobiotics could fall under the classification of Traditional Oriental Medicine as it operates using the principles of Yin and Yang.

The Roots of Oriental Medicine

Traditional Oriental medicine has its roots in China three to five thousand years ago. Several old texts have been discovered, the most famous of which is the Huang Di Nei Jing, which translates as the 'Yellow Emperor, Inner Cannon', which dates around 475-221BC and is considered the earliest medical text on Acupuncture and Chinese medicine.

This book which is laid out in a question and answer format between the mythical Yellow Emperor and six of his ministers covers such matters of health and disease and discusses the concept of Qi/Ki, the channel systems and the acupuncture points. This book is a key point of reference and an essential syllabus for acupuncture practitioners and students today. Essentially it is the bible for acupuncturists.

Throughout the centuries, other contributors have written texts and pooled their findings right up to the current age. Traditional Chinese medicine continued to be practiced and refined over the centuries and has survived to the modern age.

In China, hospitals have departments of acupuncture, herbal medicine and massage alongside departments of 'orthodox' medicine. A growing body of research studies has been produced to give traditional Oriental medicine an evidence base according to modern Western scientific protocols although some of these studies are not always given equal weight in the West.

Chinese medicine has also travelled to other countries since its beginning, particularly in Korea and Japan as well as other East Asian countries. In Japan, it underwent a different kind of development and refinement – a trait typical of the Japanese, if we look at their careful development and refinement of cars and electronics such as Sony and Toyota.

In Japan, acupuncture techniques became gentler and the needle quality was improved as seen by the Japanese needle brand of Seirin, a finer, higher quality and more expensive brand of acupuncture needle which can be less painful to insert.

Traditional Oriental Medicine is closely related to Taoism – a religious, philosophical and ritual tradition that emphasizes living in harmony with the 'Tao'. The Tao can be described as the 'way of life' or the natural order of nature. The Tao is described in the ancient text 'the Tao te Ching' written by the famous Chinese philosopher Laozi sometime in the 4th or 5th century BC.

Amazing Innovations of the Ancient Chinese

Sometimes, Traditional medicine is dismissed as being archaic, a throw-back to ancient medicine that should have gone the way of the dodo much like the four humors theory of medicine (blood, yellow bile, black bile and phlegm) as accredited to Hippocrates, the originator of the Hippocratic oath – *'first do no harm'*.

It is an easy argument to make of a time that did not have the technology to see germs and viruses, let alone understand DNA strands. However, what is sometimes overlooked is that the ancient Chinese were an extremely technologically advanced civilization and were responsible for a great many innovations.

It was the Chinese that first utilized paper money. They developed technology such as the compass and undertook long sea journeys as far back as the early 15th century to the East coast of Africa in large mega ships that were estimated to be twice the size of the largest European ships that came a hundred years later.

They were attributed with developing the first seismometer to detect the direction an earthquake was coming from. There are other innovations like gunpowder, fireworks, tea, toilet paper and wood block printing – the precursor to the printing press.

There are a great many technological innovations but it is also within the range of healthcare, that the ancient Chinese made some discoveries. For example, it is generally accepted that vaccination or inoculation – the introduction of a weak form of the disease to stimulate the human body to develop an immunity to be able to fight off specific epidemics was a product of modern scientific medicine.

In the 1880s, the small pox inoculation was promoted by Edward Jenners in England and was taken up by the government of the time.

However, the technique of inoculation was also recorded as being practiced in China during the song dynasty in the tenth century. The story goes that following the death of his eldest son to the disease, Prime Minister Wang Don sought to prevent the same fate happening to others. He summoned physicians and specialists from all over China, whereby a Taoist monk introduced the technique. In the 16th century, there were other reports of inoculation being practiced.

In the classical text 'the Inner Cannon of the Yellow Emperor, there are certainly indications that the ancient Chinese were carrying out autopsies and studying the internal organs based on diagrams. including an understanding of the circulation of the blood system.

It is worth bearing in mind, ancient China's contribution to civilisation before we start to dismiss their system of traditional medicine as being out of date or primitive. The ancient Chinese were innovators and scientists and they were able to marry a philosophical understanding of man and nature with a pragmatic approach to the world and to health and disease.

Introduction of Acupuncture to the West

In the summer of 1971, New York columnist James Reston was in China covering Richard Nixon's iconic visit to China. During the trip, James was taken severely ill with acute appendicitis and he needed to have emergency surgery carried out in at hospital.

Unfortunately, after the operation, he suffered from intense post-operative pain for which no relief could be gained from painkillers. At this time, he was offered acupuncture and moxibustion treatment, which helped relieve some of his discomfort. He wrote about his experiences and then as relations opened up between Communist China and Capitalist America, unusual reports started coming out of China in the 1970s regarding this mysterious old medicine called acupuncture.

Westerners were amazed with stories of open-heart surgery being carried out with acupuncture and no anesthesia. They were treated to pictures of Chinese men with their chests opened up surrounded by doctors in gowns all apparently pain free thanks to the power of the acupuncture needle or happily chatting to the doctors after the surgery.

With all of these reports and Reston's experience, a certain amount of hype was created on the magic of acupuncture, which helped launch Oriental Medicine into the West at a time when the West was ready and willing for it.

It should be noted, that things are not always as they seem. Over time, some of the Chinese doctors that participated in these exhibitions began to share certain bits of knowledge – that the patients would be pre-selected depending on their higher tolerance to pain - that some patients would be given a combination of painkillers, which may or may not have had an influence on the pain - that there would usually be an anesthetist standing by in case the acupuncture didn't work.

These facts do take away some of the gloss off these events, but not the result - Chinese medicine had gained widespread attention in the West. This was not Chinese medicine's first introduction to the West, but it was perhaps its most sensational. One of the first individuals recognized to bring acupuncture to the West was the Frenchman George Soulie de Morant.

George Soulie de Morant, 1878-1955 lived for many years in China working for a bank and as part of the French diplomatic corps. A scholar and writer, he learnt Chinese and developed an interest in Chinese medicine.

In 1899, he was sent to China. According to sources, his interest in acupuncture was created when he saw its use during a cholera outbreak. He took this opportunity to study under popular teachers at the time. On a side note, the type of acupuncture Morant would have experienced would have been different to the more modern system of acupuncture today developed by Mao's People Republic of China which aimed to make acupuncture and Chinese medicine more structured and standardized in line with Western systems of medicine.

On his return in 1917, Morant promoted acupuncture by authoring a number of articles for scientific journals and also worked in a hospital department for a while along with translating various Chinese works.

He combined his experiences and wrote an epic textbook called 'L' Acuponcture Chinoise or' 'Chinese Acupuncture', in which he discussed concepts as the theory of energy and circulation in the channel system. This unique book, laid out in complex detail the teaching of the channel pathways, and the acupuncture points and the best methods to treat various diseases.

Today, this text has fallen out of common use for acupuncture students, but it is still a text worth studying for the serious acupuncture practitioner. For his contributions, Morant was nominated for the Nobel Prize in 1950.

In the preceding years, there have been many great contributors to the growth of Traditional Oriental Medicine in the West. Some are well known – authors, academics, teachers, organizers of new schools and systems. But there are a far greater many contributors living daily lives practicing from small clinics or their own homes helping people around them with problems and sharing their knowledge and skill quietly in their local neighborhoods or with fellow practitioners. There may be one in your local neighborhood right now that you haven't yet met.

Eastern Mind Meets Modern West – Yin Meets Yang

One of the biggest obstacles to the appreciation of traditional oriental medicine is the mindset that new is better and the old should be made obsolete. In the last hundred years, the world has speeded up with incredible advancements in technology as well as medicine.

We can travel the planet in a day. We can communicate instantaneously with people thousands of miles away whilst sitting on our sofas. We have advancements in food production, sanitation as well as the explosion of medical pharmaceuticals such as antibiotics and steroids. We have more diagnostic tests such as MRI scans, ultrasound and other procedures such as organ transplants, keyhole surgery, and IVF.

If we continue along this path, perhaps the goal is that we can envision a Star Trek-like future regarding medicine, whereby a scanner can scan the body and detect even the slightest abnormality and another scanner or hyper syringe can fix it within minutes. Already, we are light years ahead of the ancient Chinese or any other Ancient civilisation, or so we think.

I believe that we are still a long way off from achieving this. The reason is that modern medicine seeks to break down and compartmentalize the person into separate parts and study each part as though it is independent of the whole, which includes the individual's life experiences and emotions.

Modern medicine, and in particular pharmaceutical medicine, works from a premise that the human body is incapable of healing or regulating itself.

Modern Western medicine's greatest strength is in the treatments of acute diseases. However, it has a very simplistic approach to disease ranging from its *slash and burn* approach to cancer or its over-dependence on pharmaceuticals for every other disease.

Fundamentally, the problem with most pharmaceuticals is that firstly they are suppressive in their nature. And secondly, they are alien to the body and always come with side effects - some mild and tolerable, but others are as extreme as the problem they are trying to stop. For example, some cancer drugs may increase the chances of other types of cancer developing as a potential side effect.

Unfortunately, we have seen the rise of chronic conditions like diabetes, asthma, and other autoimmune diseases. Heart disease and cancer are the two biggest premature killers of humans.

Despite the 'war on cancer', cancer rates still stubbornly refuse to fall and certain types of cancer have actually increased. Another epidemic is that of depression. Antidepressant use is becoming common and we have the seriously questionable practice today of children being prescribed mood altering drugs such as Ritalin. This practice should send alarm bells ringing but it doesn't.

Obesity levels are at a disturbing level in the USA and are increasing in the UK, which brings with it all types of health problems. For much of our history, the problems of poverty, poor sanitation, clean food, malnutrition, infectious diseases and epidemics were the biggest health threats.

Now today, the problem is too much food of poor nutritious quality - much of it is processed with high levels of carbohydrates and sugar, or grown in severely depleted soil that does not even have half the nutrients that were present 50 years ago due to over farming and aggressive land use.

Fortunately, sanitation, a reduction in malnutrition and the use of antibiotics have reduced the incidences of infectious disease which had been declining for decades as social conditions improved.

We are no longer plagued with outbreaks of plague, typhoid fever, scarlet fever, cholera or tuberculosis (TB), although TB has been on the rise amongst some of the homeless and incoming refugees in recent years.

Instead we have increasing levels of autoimmune disease – asthma, diabetes, neurological illness such as multiple sclerosis (MS), inflammatory bowel illness such as colitis and Crohns disease, arthritis as well as general allergies.

It could be argued that we have traded one set of health problems for another. Unfortunately, these chronic diseases are not curable by Western medicine which does has the power to understand what is going wrong but not why or how to fix it, other than the long-term use of drugs designed to suppress the symptoms.

For various common conditions, some modern treatments are simply not effective. Others are very effective, but have uncomfortable side effects. It is for this reason that many people start to look for solutions to their healthcare concerns in the Complementary or Alternative Medicine (CAM) arena.

There are people that attack CAM and anyone who uses it, but they ignore two facts - (1) that people basically want relief from their suffering and will turn to whoever can provide it. (2) That these people are not getting adequate relief from conventional orthodox medicine despite what the *studies* and *research* say and that they move to CAM as a final choice as opposed to a first course of action.

Another factor is the growing dissatisfaction with the medical system particularly in the UK, which is becoming dangerously overstretched and runs more like a factory conveyer belt than a caring profession. We are allotted 5 minute appointments with a tired overworked GP, who gets impatient if we start to run overtime.

When we go to a doctor we go in expecting his or her full attention and a relationship of trust. The increasing reality is that they are overworked and over-stretched and you are simply one face among hundreds that week. Will they remember you if you cross them walking down the street?

On top of that is the admin and forms that they must fulfil for recording purposes. I remember one appointment with a GP where he spent the entire 5 minutes of my consultation typing down what I said onto my electronic file on his computer. I think he looked at me only once directly during the whole consultation. On the NHS, you are less likely to get an appointment on the day or even the week that you call the reception.

Most receptionists will act as gatekeepers when you call and ask you what ails you so that they can triage the importance of your call. The problem is these are not medically trained people. They are receptionists and such a decision such as triaging should not be put to them because they will lack the knowledge and may miss a significant detail.

Hospital appointments are hard to come by with long waiting lists. People have been known to die waiting months for an operation that may save them. A&E departments have horrendous wait times – where you may typically wait several hours to be seen. Maternity wards are overfilled with queues for the labour room.

Despite these stresses on the system, it is amazing that the people who work as nurses and doctors still carry on professionally and to their highest ability, but sooner or later, these pressures on the system will become too much.

The downside to all this is that a great many people don't develop a good relationship with their doctors, which can be essential for true healing. Some consultants can be quite arrogant with godlike attitudes forgetting that they are there to serve the patient, not the other way around. If mistakes occur as they will in any system that is over-burdened, these mistakes are covered up and never acknowledged. Sometimes, even the patient will be blamed for their health problems.

Another casualty is choice. Perhaps you don't want your 90-year-old grandmother to undergo chemotherapy which may prolong her life a few more months but carry with it horrible side effects, yet she may be pushed into it.

Perhaps you want to explore the possibility that a health condition can be helped with diet or other types of complementary therapies instead of being prescribed another drug to go with all the others. However, if you voice these questions or refuse accepted treatment protocols your concerns may fall on deaf ears. Also, because many modern health problems are chronic but not necessarily life threatening, there is only so much aid you will get from a doctor for them.

The greatest strength of conventional medicine is in acute care particularly accident and emergency as well as the diagnosis and examination of problems. If you are run over in the street by a car, have a burst appendix, or a serious acute infection, a medical center is the place for you not an acupuncturist.

If you have recurrent, persistent unusual symptoms for a long period of time or strange bleeding, then a medical doctor is trained to differentiate these different symptoms into a suspected diagnosis and will have access to sophisticated equipment that may help investigate what they problem may be.

However, it is in the treatment of chronic illness, the options are mostly restricted to the long-term use of suppressive drugs which may not always work and is why many people turn to therapies like acupuncture and herbal medicine at this point.

Doctors will rarely talk about lifestyle factors that can improve some conditions naturally such as the types of foods you eat, how much to eat or how you prepare your foods. Nor will they consider the role of emotions and stress as a trigger for the onset of specific diseases. If you do discuss emotions, the chances are you will be prescribed an antidepressant or diazepam.

It should be considered incredible that modern medicine will simply admit that the cause of many diseases is *unknown* or is due to *genetic factors*, which doesn't really mean anything. The problem is that too much time is spent on studying disease but not on studying health. It is the equivalent of studying how someone can become rich just by studying the life, mindset and habits of a poor person.

What does being healthy mean? What is the best way to live a healthy life? Herein lies the necessity of caring about diet, of emotions, of using your body the way nature intended, of challenging your body and spirit and occasionally pushing it to its limit, but not beyond. On this path, is the necessity to pay attention to how your body is doing on a day to day basis and of listening to the messages it is telling you.

Oriental medicine and in particular acupuncture is at its heart very simple. It is based on common sense and the careful observation of nature and of the human body. For example, if something is cold, it needs to be warmed. If something is blocked, its needs to be cleared. What makes acupuncture so relevant in the modern age is that it requires us to listen closely to the messages the body is telling us.

This may go against the message of society where we are encouraged to leave the business of our bodies to professionals. We are so busy nowadays. Work, family, career, money, appointments, and commuting occupies our days. Entertainment – TV, music, social media and the internet takes care of the rest. Our lives are stimulated full, far beyond what our ancestors would have known. Time seems to flow faster and it has become the new norm.

We are perhaps not aware, that while this stimulates our lives more, it also drains us. It is essential that we learn to listen to our bodies more. Our bodies do have self-healing powers and though we can help the process along, it is our bodies that heal us when we are injured.

Our bodies repair bones. It is our bodies that make babies. An acupuncture needle from the hand of a practitioner simply stimulates our body's own healing response when it is unable to do it by itself. Oriental medicine seeks to see the body and life experience as a whole rich tapestry rather than to break it down in a mechanistic way. Just because one section of the body such as the bowel or pancreas or ovary is diseased does not mean that the whole body is not involved in some holistic way.

Prevention better than cure

In Veith's translation of the Yellow Emperors Cannon of Internal Medicine (Huangdi Neijing), there is this passage: –

> "The sages did not treat those who were already ill, they instructed those who were not yet ill. To administer medicine to diseases which have already developed is comparable to the behaviour of those persons who begin to dig a well after they have become thirsty and of those who begin to cast weapons after they have already engaged in battle. Would these actions not be too late?"

This extract emphasizes the importance of preventative treatment and following a healthy balanced lifestyle in tune with nature (or the Tao). Many diseases take time to develop and obvious symptoms may not show up until the disease has become more fixed.

This sums up very well the problem of patients with advanced disease. By the time we see them, it may already be too late. The disease process is far more advanced and in many cases the best we can offer is symptomatic improvements such as reducing pain, digestive discomfort, and improving anxiety and stress or dealing with the side effects of pharmaceutical drugs like chemotherapy or post-operative recovery.

Perhaps, the best time would be to have started treating these people in the early stages of their illness when they first started getting symptoms or before. Of course, it is easier to say this with hindsight and no guarantees that any therapy can prevent complex health problems.

However, acupuncture treatment and indeed many complementary therapies can enhance life, reduce stress, improve bodily function and boost the immune system and has the potential to be a good preventative measure.

This is the reason why such therapies needs be promoted more and to become more of an accepted mainstream medical system. One of acupuncture's potential strengths is that it may have the power to keep a person in balanced health if used frequently. However, proof of this is still dependent on more scientific studies being carried out.

One example is an elderly patient arriving with widespread arthritis and bone deformity through their body suffering from severe pain and taking a cocktail of pharmaceuticals. An acupuncture and moxibustion treatment may temporary remove the pain, but it will come back because the underlying problem is well entrenched.

The patient can continue to have repeated treatments but this can be expensive. It may perhaps be more beneficial If the patient started a gentle form of tai chi specifically for elderly people and if they administered self-moxibustion treatment daily and had regular hot baths.

By doing this, they can encourage the flow of Ki-energy and blood, improve circulation and reduce the stagnation which causes the pain. However, this process can take months, perhaps years and requires effort on the part of the patient.

If at the same time, they continued with regular acupuncture treatments, the pain may be able to be reduced or lessened to a manageable level and that person may be able to gain more mobility again, improving the quality of their life.

If the person also experimented with reducing food with inflammatory properties, by cutting out fried foods, red meats, dairy and also increasing their intake of fresh vegetables and oily fish, that would also help. If the person practiced meditation or mindfulness, this may also help moderate the mental aspects of their suffering.

Yet imagine if a middle-aged person, who with the early signs of arthritis setting in, was to undertake these changes in their 50s, the trajectory of their life and old age could be much altered. Positive changes can be taken at any time in life. Of course, the earlier the better and there is no better time than today.

204

409

CONCLUSION

In this book, we have looked at some of the history, principles and theories behind Traditional Oriental Medicine. We have looked at factors that can influence our health like how we use our bodies, how to eat and how to counteract the harmful effects of tension and stress. We have looked at simple common sense living habits. But the most important thing to take away from this book is that of responsibility.

Responsibility for our bodies, our lives and our destiny. Our bodies are the vessels that carry us through our lives. They come in different shapes and sizes and have all sorts of different strengths or weakness, which we must learn to figure out.

Fundamentally, our body is the vessel for our spirit. It is our spirit that seeks out, grows and thrives from the various experiences of life. It is our job to give our spirit the experience it needs for a fulfilling life. Ultimately, we are responsible for looking after our bodies by our daily life practices and choices on how we treat and fuel them.

We have the power to take control of our lives

It is this objective that powers the philosophy of this book. We have to take responsibility for our health. There are things we can learn to do that can help us and possibly stop some problems from occurring in the future.

For example, if we eat too much red meat - introduce more white meats, fish or vegetables into our diet. If we eat too much fried foods - eat less and instead eat more vegetables or wholegrains.

If we drink too much alcohol, explore our drinking habits and why we need to drink so much and of course - drink less. If we smoke - stop, smoke moderately or on special occasions. If we overeat - eat less.

If we live or work in an intensely stressful environment which is seriously impacted our health and wellbeing – make plans to find alternative employment or change our working environment.

If our lives are unhappy - find ways to bring joy into it daily. If something in our daily life is slowly killing us, it is up to us to deal with it before it actually does. It is up to us to take proactive steps to improve our health.

The power is in our hands. To follow life enhancing practices whilst we are healthy is the equivalent of digging the well long before we run out of water. Such things require discipline to create new habits.

Discipline is a good way to build willpower and to break addictions to cravings. This book has shown some simple pro-active steps we can take to improve our health

There are many components to good health such as the way we use our bodies, the power of emotions, our purpose and place in society. By considering these factors, we take a *holistic* view of ourselves and our place in the universe.

There is a lot more information that this book doesn't contain, but I hope that this book will have enough for the reader to consider and go on for now.

For more information, visit the author's website and blog at

www.johndixonacupuncture.co.uk

REFERENCES

Chinese Acupuncture. George Soulie de Morant. Paradigm Publications. Brookline, 1972.

Walking in Roman Culture, Timothy M. O'Sullivan. Cambridge University press 2011.

Geoff Pike. The Power of Chi. 1985. Bay Books.

Veith I. Yellow Emperor's Classic of Internal Medicine: Chapters 1-34. 1992. University of California Press.

Shakespeare, William. Hamlet. Oxford University Press 1987.

Qigong: Assessment of Immunological Parameters following a Qigong Training Program. Juan M. Manzaneque et al. 2004; 10(6): CR264-270 www.MedSciMonit.com

Impact of Medical Qigong on quality of life, fatigue, mood and inflammation in cancer patients: a randomized trial. B Oh, P. Butow, B. Mullan, S. Clarke, P. Beale, N. Pavlakis, E. Kothe, L. Lam, D. Rosenthal. Annals of Oncology 21: 608-614. 2009

Factors associated with "Ikigai" among members of a public temporary employment agency for seniors (Silver Human Resources Centre) in Japan; gender differences. K. Shirai et al, 27th February 2006. *Health and Quality of Life Outcomes* 2006, 4:12 doi:10.1186/1477-7525-4-12. BioMed Central Ltd.

Were Ötzi the iceman's tattoos an early form of 'acupuncture'? Sarah Griffiths, 28th October 2013. Daily Mail. Accessed 1st February 2017 http://www.dailymail.co.uk/sciencetech/article-2478420/Were-tzi-icemans-tattoos-early-form-acupuncture-Scientists-believe-5-000-year-old-skin-etchings-therapeutic.html

Macrobiotics: Yesterday and Today. RE Kotzsch, Ph.D. Japan Publications, Inc. 1985, Tokyo and New York

The Only Two Causes of All Diseases, by Toru Abo 2013, published by Babel Press USA

A Shiatsu Story: Tokujiro Namikoshi Remembered. Kensen Saito. Massage Bodywork Magazine, Feb/March 2001. Associated Bodywork and Massage Professionals.

http://www.massagetherapy.com/articles/index.php/article_id/113/A-Shiatsu-Story Accessed 23rd February 2017

Is There a Role for Postmortem Acupuncture? By Jeffrey Dann. Volume 19 Number 55. July 2012. North American Journal of Oriental Medicine, pg 19

Toru Abo. Your Immune Revolution and Healing your Healing Power: Achieve Longevity by Controlling the Hypothermia and Hypoxia! Babel Press 2013

Minimalism: Reuters.com June 20th 2016 'Less is more as Japanese minimalist movement grows' Megumi Lim (accessed 30/10/16).

Seven Taoist Masters. A Folk Novel of China. Eva Wong. Shambhala Classics. Boston & London 2004

Dietary restriction in mice beginning at 1 year of age: effect on life-span and spontaneous cancer incidence. R. Weindruch & RL Walford. Science, 12 March 1982. Vol. 215, Issue 4538, pp 1415-1418. DOI: 10.1126/science.7063854

A Calory-Restricted Diet Decreases Brain Iron Accumulation and preserves Motor Performance in Old Rhesus Monkeys. EK Eastman et al. Journal of Neuroscience 9 June 2010, 30 (23) 7940-7947; DOI: https://doi.org/10.1523/JNEUROSCI.10.2010

Michiyo Mori 'The Age of No Eating'. https://www.youtube.com/watch?v=MkHz4kk9mEQ. Accessed 1st December 2017

Confucius. The Analects. 1997 Chichung Huang. Oxford University Press. New York.

Picture Credits

Model for Exercise Pictures: Eitaro Hamano

Acupuncture Picture: Copyright: <a href='https://www.123rf.com/profile_sheeler'>sheeler / 123RF Stock Photo</a>

Channel Pathway: Copyright: <a href='http://www.123rf.com/profile_peterhermesfurian'>peterhermesfurian / 123RF Stock Photo</a>

Image of Discobolus: Copyright: <a href='http://www.123rf.com/profile_copestello'>copestello / 123RF Stock Photo</a>

Hand Massage: Copyright: <a href='http://www.123rf.com/profile_imarly'>imarly / 123RF Stock Photo</a>

Congee picture: Copyright: <a href='http://www.123rf.com/profile_jreika'>jreika / 123RF Stock Photo</a>

Yin Yang Symbol: Copyright: Image ID: 12453011 www.123rf.com

Link for Moxa. Copyright: <a href='https://www.123rf.com/profile_sheeler'>sheeler / 123RF Stock Photo</a>

Image link meditation Chinese woman lotus position: Copyright: <a href='http://www.123rf.com/profile_cardmaverick'>cardmaverick / 123RF Stock Photo</a>

Slumped on sofa Picture: Copyright: <a href='https://www.123rf.com/profile_ximagination'>ximagination / 123RF Stock Photo</a>

Link slumped in office (caucasian). Copyright: <a href='https://www.123rf.com/profile_andreypopov'>andreypopov / 123RF Stock Photo</a>

Chinese woman seiza attribution link: Copyright: <a href='http://www.123rf.com/profile_cardmaverick'>cardmaverick / 123RF Stock Photo</a>

Reflexology Diagram:Link: Reflexology. Copyright: <a href='http://www.123rf.com/profile_vampy1'>vampy1 / 123RF Stock Photo</a>

Morning Stretch: Copyright: <a href='https://www.123rf.com/profile_leungchopan'>leungchopan / 123RF Stock Photo</a>

Image of Onsen, drawn by S. Kawai.

Image of boy slumped on sofa. Copyright: <a href='https://www.123rf.com/profile_mdilsiz'>mdilsiz / 123RF Stock Photo</a>

Image of kyphosis. Copyright: <a href='https://www.123rf.com/profile_hfsimaging'>hfsimaging / 123RF Stock Photo</a

Printed in Poland
by Amazon Fulfillment
Poland Sp. z o.o., Wrocław

51908813R00125